The Obesity Epidemic
and its Management

The Obesity Epidemic and its Management

A textbook for primary healthcare professionals on the understanding, management and treatment of obesity

Terry Maguire BSc, PhD, FCPP, FPSNI, MRPharmS (Hon Member), FPSI
Community Pharmacist, Proprietor of Maguire Pharmacies, Belfast, UK

David Haslam MB BS, DGM
Chair of the National Obesity Forum (NOF), London, UK and Professor at the Faculty of Health and Social Care, Robert Gordon University, Aberdeen, UK and General Practitioner, Senior Partner at Watton Place Clinic, UK

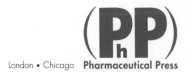

London • Chicago **Pharmaceutical Press**

Published by the Pharmaceutical Press
An imprint of RPS Publishing

1 Lambeth High Street, London SE1 7JN, UK
1559 St Paul Avenue, Gurnee, IL 60031, USA

© Pharmaceutical Press 2010

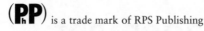 is a trade mark of RPS Publishing

RPS Publishing is the publishing organisation of the
Royal Pharmaceutical Society of Great Britain

First published 2010

Typeset by Type Study, Scarborough, UK
Printed in Great Britain by TJ International, Padstow, Cornwall

ISBN 978 0 85369 786 2

A catalogue record for this book is available from the British Library.

FSC
Mixed Sources
Product group from well-managed
forests and other controlled sources
Cert no. SGS-COC-2482
www.fsc.org
© 1996 Forest Stewardship Council

Contents

Preface

Obesity is a highly visible public health problem. We see it on the high streets, in the shopping malls and in the restaurants and, as the numbers in the population classified as overweight or obese become more common, we sadly seem to be getting immune to it. But becoming immune cannot be a solution; complacency will only serve to further increase the costs of too many people carrying too many pounds of unnecessary body fat for too many years of their lives. For developed nations, and for many developing nations too, obesity and its consequences are possibly the biggest public health problem they face as we reach the end of the first decade of the 21st century. Cigarette smoking still remains a significant cost to health but obesity is quickly outpacing smoking as the number one cause of morbidity and mortality; in addition it proves to be a considerable resource burden on already overstretched healthcare systems. In 40 years time if nothing is done, and the 20% of the population who are now obese turn into 50% of the population, then the consequences will indeed be dire as our healthcare systems, as currently constituted, will simply become bankrupt trying to cope.

Yet, since humans must eat to live, obesity, and its resolution, has proved to be a stubborn public health challenge. For most, getting fat is seen as a natural part of life; adding a few pounds year by year is the expectation of the public. Often weight gain and the change in body shape associated with it is seen as a cosmetic problem rather than a threat to health. As a consequence, motivation to change lifestyle to lose weight for health reasons is often lacking. Ironically weight loss for cosmetic reasons has been turned into a global multi-billion dollar industry with an emphasis on weight loss methods that have more to do with vanity and commerce than improving health. There is herein an interesting paradox. For example, health gyms in the US are now more popular than they have ever been, yet this is at a time when 50% of individuals in the US population are moving towards an obese classification in their BMI measurements.[1]

A solution to the obesity problem, and a reduction in its consequential morbidity and mortality, will only be arrived at through the concerted efforts of governments, other agencies and businesses, communities, the family unit and individuals themselves. It will call for appropriate government regulation, greater societal engagement and improved individual understanding of the problem and the assumption of greater personal responsibility for health. Indeed, in the UK, this was the recommendation of the Wanless Report in 2004[2] which appreciated the consequences should no action be taken. This will not be easy to achieve and it will take time.

At government level there will need to be a greater appetite to tackle those elements within the food industry that are failing to take responsibility for their role in the creation and sustaining of this public health crisis. Already there have been attempts for improved food standards, guidelines on food consumption, better food labelling and improved standards for advertising of high-calorie foods to children. But often these have been voluntary agreements that in practice have not been adhered too as companies favour shareholders' interests over the interests of public health. Certainly the fast food industries and supermarkets share some of the blame for a fatter nation and, whereas they have taken some small steps in accepting responsibility, these steps have often been insignificant or merely tokens.

Obesity is a wider problem than the food we eat, where we buy it or where we consume it. We have in our towns and cities created environments that are assisting the rapid rise of obesity in the population. This obesogenic environment is a major contributor by denying people easy access to sufficient daily exercise. Town planning and building design needs to better understand the metabolic needs of the human body and this must become a priority in all new planning schemes.

Communities, particularly less well-off ones, need to identify their needs regarding obesity and its impact, and they need to lobby for better facilities whether this be fairly priced fresh fruit and vegetable or better, safer, open spaces for exercise. The individual too needs a better understanding of basic nutrition and as a result becomes able to make healthier choices regarding food and exercise opportunities.

This book is aimed at the primary healthcare worker: the pharmacist, the general practitioner and the practise or community nurse, and is designed to provide a basic understanding of the problem and why it has become such a major public health crisis over the past 30 years. Once we have stated the problem in Part 1, in Part 2 we consider some solutions. This understanding we hope will provide those working in primary care to support the patients and clients with whom they have day-to-day professional contact so that advice can be given that will allow individuals to make better choices in the foods they eat and the level of exercise they take. In this way it will be possible for some to avoid becoming overweight or obese. If individuals are already obese we hope to provide an understanding of what is available to support sustainable weight loss that will reduce disease risk. For some, simple lifestyle changes will be insufficient and therefore we consider other proven options such as pharmacotherapy and surgery. We also consider the complex and often confusing area of fad diets and over-the-counter slimming aids, most of which have very little basis in science but for which people are willing to pay a high price.

1. Olshansky S *et al*. A potential decline in life expectancy in the United States of America in the 21st century. *N Engl J Med* 2005; 352: 1138–1142.
2. Wanless D. *Securing Good Health for the Whole Population*. London: HM Treasury, 2004.

Terry Maguire, Belfast
David Haslam, Dunstable
January 2009

Acknowledgements

So many people have helped directly and indirectly in the production of this book that it would be impossible to acknowledge them all, so we begin with an apology for those we have missed out. Sincere thanks to our colleagues from PharmacyHealthLink, the UK charity that promotes public health through the UK's pharmacy network, particularly Miriam Armstrong and Geof Rayner for their insights and support. We also acknowledge the contributions of the women and staff of the Falls Women's Association, particularly Oonagh Marron and Brenda Downes, who helped with the Healthy Weight Challenge, the forerunner of the Coventry obesity pilot project, and the team working on the project, particularly Richard Balcon, Meera Shah and Ben from Unichem's pharmacy professional team.

About the authors

Dr Terry Maguire graduated from Queen's University, Belfast in 1980 and obtained a PhD in 1984. He is a Fellow and Past President of the Pharmaceutical Society of Northern Ireland, an Honorary Member of the Royal Pharmaceutical Society of Great Britain, Fellow of the Pharmaceutical Society of Ireland and a Fellow of the College of Pharmacy Practice. He has served on the PharmacyHealthLink (of which he was vice-chair from 2002 to 2007). He served as a member of the UK Committee on Safety of Medicines from 2002 to 2006, during which time he chaired the Working Group on Nicotine Replacement Therapy (NRT). He owns and managers two pharmacies in Belfast and is an honorary Senior Lecturer at the School of Pharmacy, The Queen's University of Belfast.

Dr David Haslam is Professor of Obesity Sciences at Robert Gordon University, Aberdeen and a GP with a special interest in obesity and cardiometabolic disease, Physician in Obesity Medicine at the Centre for Obesity Research at Luton & Dunstable Hospital, and Clinical Director of the National Obesity Forum in the UK. He took charge of formulating the guidelines for adult obesity management in primary care and produced the first primary care guidelines for the management of childhood obesity with the Royal College of Paediatrics and Child Health.

He is Chair of the charity Foundations, a Director of PCOS UK, a member of the Counterweight Board, Visiting Lecturer at Chester University and Visiting Fellow at the Bedfordshire and Hertfordshire Postgraduate Medical School.

David has authored articles that have been published widely, and speaks internationally on obesity and related diseases. His books include *Fast Facts: Obesity* with Professor Gary Wittert (Health Press, 2009) and *Fat, Gluttony and Sloth: obesity in literature, art and medicine* (Liverpool University Press, 2009).

PART 1

Problem statement

This section sets out the public health problem posed by a high percentage of overweight and obese individuals within the population.

1

Facts and figures

Introduction

Obesity is the accumulation of excess fat (adipose tissue) in the body, caused by the consumption of more calories than is necessary to provide the required energy for each day's activity, thus falling foul of the energy balance equation.[1]

Some working in this area of public health feel strongly that obesity should not be viewed as a disease; rather they feel obesity should be seen as a natural response to an unnatural environment, an environment where high-energy foods are available, on demand, with fewer calories expended in their procurement. This 'obesogenic' environment has essentially been created in developed countries through the commercial imperative and the activities of the market which, for a profit, seeks to serve and satisfy the wants and needs of the population.[2] A side-effect of the unparalleled recent advances in technology, itself essentially a good thing, has been the resultant reduction in human activity. In developing countries, as wealth increases, the 'obesogenic' environment rapidly develops and is accompanied by a surge in the percentage of the population classed as overweight and obese. This is the societal view of the obesity epidemic fixed in the wider determinants of health, such as the environment, education and individual and community empowerment, within which solutions are potentially available to address this health crisis. These solutions might include better provision of affordable quality foods, easy access to activity and a better understanding of the personal impact of an unhealthy lifestyle.

Others disagree with the societal model, arguing that obesity is indeed a medical condition. Obesity, like any other disease, needs first and foremost to be prevented but otherwise, supporters of the medical model of obesity argue, to be treated and managed.[3] In one respect, obesity is analogous, for example, to essential hypertension which, in itself, is only a risk factor for the development of other diseases such as coronary heart disease and stroke, but obesity has the 'advantage' of having obvious external manifestations to aid diagnosis.

In another respect obesity is a more complex condition, in that it is not only a primary risk factor for serious chronic disease in its own right, but also acts indirectly by adversely affecting other primary risk factors such as lipid profile, glycaemic control and blood pressure, among others. In the medical model, normalising blood pressure reduces the risk of resultant conditions and management is mainly through pharmacological intervention using therapeutic guidelines. In essential hypertension a role for lifestyle management as a prevention strategy is much simpler, and arguably less prominent, since there is perhaps less evidence of its success. Although salt intake and sedentary behaviour have gained recent prominence, the link between lifestyle and essential hypertension is much less clear than it is for obesity, thus the debate over environmental versus lifestyle or pharmacological intervention is currently raging. It seems obvious that both the societal and the medical models each have a role to play in tackling obesity. The combination of a societal and a medical approach is the only way to tackle adequately the problems associated with excess body fat and its resultant morbidity and mortality.[4]

Obesity is a serious problem but its insidious nature perhaps hides its current and future impact on human health. Indeed it has been described as 'as serious a threat as climate change' and other sources assert that world governments are focusing too much on fighting terrorism, while obesity and other 'lifestyle diseases' are killing millions more people.[5]

What is clear is that the impact of obesity as a public health problem is similar to, yet qualitatively different from, the impact of tobacco. No one needs to smoke and the health message to quit is simple, understandable and has universal agreement among health practitioners, i.e. stop smoking. Obesity is much more complex; everyone must eat. For this reason, public education, an essential component of any strategy to prevent and manage obesity, is more challenging and runs the risk of being too complex, confusing and unpalatable for public consumption. Public health messages related to obesity and its prevention therefore become more diluted by this complexity, and less effective than public health messages targeted at tobacco. The nature of public health advice regarding healthy eating and exercise can be confusing for the general population who often find it difficult to make sense of the information, and as a result fail to use it in informing lifestyle choices and decisions.

There are of course many vested interests. Obesity has itself become a huge industry with rich pickings for many competing sectors that fight for their say and their share and in doing so can, paradoxically, become detrimental to finding a solution. Unlike the tobacco problem, where the tobacco industry is easily singled out as the villain of the piece, there is more difficulty identifying the villain, or villains, in the obesity epidemic. What is the role, for example, of the food, advertising and retail industries, the commercial gym business, the weight-loss diet industry, primary care organisations, community pharmacy, local government and even the pharmaceutical industry, in shaping and promoting the current obesity problem? Each will claim to be a key part of the solution but often there is little evidence that they are, and in some cases there is evidence they are part of the problem. There are over 20 000 commercial gym businesses in the USA, yet they exist at a time when obesity is the major and expanding public health problem.[6] The weight loss or diet business is worth $11 billion annually yet the problem continues to grow and the evidence is clear that the population is getting fatter.

Even within the medical family there is a lack of consensus on how the problem can be or should be managed. There is a real tension between those who view obesity as a medical condition, keen to apply a medical model to its management and those who view obesity as a lifestyle issue and seek greater emphasis on a social approach, comprising individual, family and community responsibility.

Indeed this debate will, over time, determine how obesity comes to be managed at a societal, community and individual level. In the UK, much of the thinking about healthcare, and how it can be afforded over the next 20 years, is being based on the potential costs of managing the public health impact of type 2 diabetes, which has its origins in the current obesity epidemic.[7]

Stereotyping

In spite of increased publicity about this subject in recent years, there is seldom any sympathy offered to the obese person. Even within the caring professions, obese individuals may be treated with prejudice. A stereotype predominates our thinking: obesity is self-inflicted and results from sloth, greed and gluttony, and ill-advised personal choices. Colin Waine, professor of primary care at Sunderland, and a general practitioner with a specialist interest in obesity, tells of speaking to a group of general practitioners on the management of obesity, and when explaining how to undertake a waist measurement accurately was challenged by a colleague who asked why there was a need to measure waist circumference since 'I know a fat bastard when I see one'. Such an attitude for a primary care practitioner is unlikely to be helpful when addressing the needs of obese individuals.[8]

Obesity therefore is an interesting and challenging public health issue, with the potential to forge together the medical and societal models of public health even more than other issues have done before. This would potentially create a more comprehensive, holistic and joined-up public health approach.[9] Prevention of obesity is, without doubt, a societal matter and best tackled within the societal model of health: improved awareness of the issue, better food, more activity, etc. being pivotal. Management of obesity once it has developed might be better achieved through the medical model: behavioural support as well as pharmacological intervention. This all demands resources and it is for politicians to decide where such resources are best invested across the spectrum of factors that impact on the development of obesity. Properly and precisely targeted, the appropriate allocation of funds will reap optimal rewards.

Obesity, vanity and disease

Obesity is a major risk factor for many medical conditions; especially type 2 diabetes and coronary heart disease. It is for this reason that obesity is now identified as a major public health issue.[10] If it was not for its substantial impact on health, rather than its mere cosmetic importance, obesity would not be on the public health agenda, would remain in the glossy, vanity magazines and would be the subject of dubious commercial medical practices, as it was 30 years ago.

Of interest, considering the cosmetic aspects of obesity, is how unfashionable obesity has become in the modern era. Rubenesque nudes were invariably overweight, yet highly attractive and at this time many influential men in European society were overweight. This fashion is, like all human fashions, determined by what the rich can obtain and the rest want. In the 1700s and 1800s poverty ensured that most people were poorly nourished, and if anything were underweight. It was only the better off in society who could afford sufficient food to become overweight and obese.[11] Today, owing to the 'obesogenic' environment we all live in, those in the lower social classes are destined to be overweight or obese, whereas the more successful have the means and determination to remain thin. For this reason the cosmetic consideration – the desire to be thin – dovetails with public health policy and it would seem that the twin desires to look better and be healthier merge and therefore represent a considerable advantage to public health. Sadly there is little evidence that these twin objectives do in fact merge. It is for the better-off in society to dabble with expensive fad diets and cosmetic surgery with no proven benefit to their health, while the rest suffer their obesity, unable to make a difference.

An obesity problem is born

Using body mass index (BMI) as a measure of obesity, it is clear that from around 1980, in the UK, and 1970 in the USA, something happened that rapidly altered the epidemiology of overweight and obesity among all classes and groups within society.[12] No single issue or event was to blame for this explosion. Rather, myriad factors coincided subtly and simultaneously, and over 25 years the current obesity problem was born. The origins of the problem lie in government policies, social developments, technical innovations and cultural shifts which, in complex fashion, have conspired to create the public health problem that is obesity.

Despite the contradictory opinions regarding the status of obesity as a social, versus a medical, condition, the World Health Organization (WHO) has already designated obesity as a disease, and its prevalence to be of epidemic proportions.[12] Obesity and related conditions fall into the category of ill-health defined by WHO as non-communicable diseases (NCDs) and avoidable chronic diseases. Obesity was listed as a disease within the International Classification of Diseases following a 1997 WHO consultation.[12] It is now formally defined as a disease of a 'classic' type, being a physiological debilitation and malfunction. However WHO is keen to point out that obesity is also a lifestyle disorder, having social and psychological ramifications, and thus connotations for management.

Causes of obesity

The development and prevalence of obesity is complex and multifactorial, involving psychology, hormones, lifestyle and environmental issues as well as hereditary factors. Since a genetic basis is far from clear, in simple terms, obesity, for the average individual, results from consumption of too many calories compared with the number expended through physical activity over a prolonged period of time.

The WHO[12] asserts that obesity is not just an indication of imbalanced nutrition and reduced physical activity but of a change in ways of living: an inappropriate intake of energy for the lifestyle that is followed. 'Western' diets have moved irrevocably towards high consumption of saturated fats, salt and refined carbohydrates, in the context of low consumption of fruit and vegetables.

Dieting?

The 'calories-in-versus-calories-out' energy balance equation is the model that currently steers health policy in the management of obesity. Yet this simplistic approach may be erroneous and might be contributing to the problem. To create a nation of calorie counters who are constantly on weight reduction diets appears to be unhelpful, and over the past 30 years it has patently failed. It might be, as Geoffrey Cannon and Hetty Einzig claimed in their 1984 book (updated in 2008), that 'dieting makes you fat'.[13] Moving away from calorie-reducing dieting as a means of dealing with obesity might appear counterintuitive but, according to recent evidence, could be a positive step. Government policy supports such a move, recommending not eating (cutting out of the diet) a Danish pastry and a chocolate bar each day, thereby reducing daily calories by 600 kcal; this will lead to effective and sustained weight reduction over time.[14] This energy deficiency, when coupled with an increase in daily activity, is all that might be necessary to return the population to pre-1980 weight profiles. However, it is unlikely to be this simple, given that it has taken developed nations hundreds of years to get to this point but developing nations seem to be rapidly adopting Western lifestyles, and suffering the consequences in a much shorter timeframe.[3]

Doing the sums

Small, daily excesses in calories, as little as 50 kcal per day, can lead to large accumulation of fat deposits over a number of years. This excess can occur through an increase in energy intake (eating too much calorie-dense foods) or a reduction in energy expenditure (too little physical activity) or both.

The National Audit Office[1] concluded that the prevalence of obesity:

- increases with age
- is more prevalent among lower socioeconomic and lower-income groups, with a particularly strong social-class gradient in women
- is more prevalent among certain ethnic groups, particularly African Caribbean and Pakistani women
- is a problem across all regions in England but shows some important regional variations.

Dietary intake

Large meal-portion sizes, consumption of foods high in fat and sugar and excess intake of soft drinks are all associated with weight gain. During the past 50 years, there has been a significant increase in the fat content of the British diet. In 1890 the percentage of calories appearing in the diet as fat was 15%; in 1990 this figure was 42%.[15] High-fat diets and frequent snacks contribute to obesity, since they reduce the conscious recognition that food has been eaten or, put another way, this pattern of eating is less likely to trigger satiety signals and stop the person eating. The fact is that fat is less satiating compared with carbohydrate.[16] Dis-inhibition has been identified in many obese people and this results in overeating. Paradoxically, a high fat intake may result in overeating to obtain enough carbohydrate to maintain glycogen stores that are much smaller than fat stores.[13] This explains why after a good meal there is always room left for dessert.

There seem to be surprisingly few good studies on diet and obesity but Bolton-Smith and Woodward[17] looked at the diet of 11 600 Scottish men and women and showed that those who got the highest percentage of their energy from carbohydrates were much less likely to be obese compared with those who derived much of their calories from fat. It is known that an inappropriate diet in pregnancy will lead to the formation of neural and metabolic pathways in the fetus that already predispose the unborn child to obesity and insulin resistance and that this effect lasts for generations.

Fast foods and processed foods that lack good nutritional properties are associated with obesity and have been assessed in the CARDIA study.[18] Weight gain and insulin resistance were found in people who ate fast food frequently, suggesting an increase in risk of type 2 diabetes. Eating frequency also plays a part in development of obesity. Serum cholesterol concentration is lower when people eat several small meals per day compared with a few large meals. The mean glucose concentration is also lowered when meals are frequent, raising the possibility of differences in insulin secretion associated with meal size.

Physical activity

Lifestyle has changed significantly in the past 100 years. In the UK, a quarter of both men and women live sedentary lifestyles. The sedentary levels increase with age and are highest (37%) in the unskilled socioeconomic groups and lowest (17%) in professional groups. The incidence of obesity and, as a consequence, its impact on health, is more significant in lower socioeconomic groups and reflects a common theme that the less well off are more likely to be unhealthy.

Age

Adults normally put on weight as they age at an average rate of around 1 kg per year. Critical periods in life appear to be associated with development of obesity.[1] Fetal nutrition has an effect on later growth and the likelihood of obesity. This appears to be a result of fatness and energy regulation. Breastfed babies are less likely to be obese in adulthood, and breastfeeding mothers are more likely to regain their figures after the birth. Breastfed infants, compared with bottle-fed, have a natural tendency to drop down the weight percentile chart at around 8 weeks in recognition of a plentiful supply of food rendering it unnecessary to over-indulge. The misinterpretation of this as failure to thrive, and the unwise 'topping-up' of these children with bottle milk is a major driver towards future obesity. Infants, especially those born prematurely, who are overfed and who experience a rapid growth in infancy are more likely to become obese adults. Rapid weight gain around the ages of 5–7 years alongside the development of new behaviour patterns can be associated with an increased risk of obesity in later life, even if this fat is lost in the short term.

In adolescence and during teenage years, independence from the family unit is often associated with irregular meals, changing food habits, and a reduction in physical activity. These changes are often associated with weight gain and are a good predictor of obesity in later life. Women, when co-habiting with a man, can gain weight since portion sizes tend to increase in line with her partner's intake. In addition the 'pill' and possible pregnancies can also induce weight gain. Furthermore, the menopause tends to be associated with a susceptibility to weight gain, particularly around the abdomen, because of hormonal changes. The elderly have unique risk factors, as they tend to suffer from sarcopenic obesity; a reduction in muscle mass because of reduced activity, alongside an increase in body fat. In this way, all stages of life, as we age, can contribute to increasing weight.

Social class

Children born to obese parents have more than double the risk of adult obesity regardless of childhood weight. Men have a higher tendency to be overweight while obesity is more common in women. There is an inverse relationship between socioeconomic status and obesity especially among women. Socioeconomic factors understandably play a role in weight control. Eating habits and type of diet can depend on knowledge and educational status, the foods available, the perceived cost of healthy foods compared with fast and convenience foods, and family mealtime routines. The most easily affordable foods are usually higher in fat and energy density, compounded by the fact that individuals with scarcer financial resources might spend more time in sedentary activities, such as watching television.

In the developed world, deprivation is associated with a lower consumption of healthier foods, for example, a 50% lower intake of fruit and vegetables compared with higher social groups. In addition there is less access to and participation in sport.

Studies have demonstrated differences in obesity between social classes. In social classes 1 and 2, the prevalence of obesity for women in 1994 was 12% and 14% respectively, in contrast to a rate of 22% and 21% in women in classes 4 and 5.[19] Obesity is also linked to educational status; women with no educational status attaining a mean BMI of 26.7 kg/m^2 compared with 24.6 kg/m^2 in those educated to 'A' level and above.[19] In England 18.7% of managerial and professional women are designated obese compared with 29.1% of women in less well-paid jobs.

Ethnic origin

Ethnic origin is an important factor. African-American and Mexican-American individuals have the highest rate of obesity in the US. Migration studies have shown an increased risk of obesity in urban environments and with Westernised lifestyles. The reason is thought to be underlying genetic predisposition, which becomes overt on exposure to unhealthy diets and lifestyles. Certain groups, such as the Pima Indians of South Dakota, and the Nauru Islanders have suffered from the change in their native environment, transforming their status from lean and healthy to predominantly obese and having chronic illness: 45% of the population of Nauru have type 2 diabetes.[16] The UK provides evidence that migrating away from traditional habits and lifestyles to new, unaccustomed ones is a cause of obesity. Second-generation descendants of migrants tend to adopt native British patterns of food consumption – increasing dietary fat and reducing fruit and vegetable intake.[1] It is important for pharmacists and other healthcare professionals who deal with different ethnic groups to be aware of the greater risk they have, and to manage them accordingly.

Medical issues

Certain physical disorders and medical conditions are associated with a tendency to obesity. Insulin resistance, as found in type 2 diabetes and polycystic ovary syndrome is associated with weight gain, and such individuals will lose only 50% of the weight lost on any given regime compared with their counterparts. Hypothyroidism, Cushing's syndrome, growth hormone and testosterone deficiency, insulinoma, and hypothalamic lesions are also linked with excess weight. Genetic disorders such as Prader-Willi syndrome, and the rare leptin deficiency condition invariably leads to obesity. People with Down's syndrome, and other physical or mental disabilities have a greater chance of being obese, and those with schizophrenia and other serious mental health problems are also predisposed to obesity and consequent cardiometabolic conditions.[20]

Cigarette smoking is associated with a lower body weight and smoking cessation is associated with weight gain for two reasons. Firstly, there is an adjustment in liver metabolism that is associated with basic metabolic rate (BMR). Over a few weeks there is a loss of enzymes that contribute to a reduction in BMR. This is associated with an increase, on average, of 2–3 kg. Secondly, there is a return or improvement in taste and smell on stopping smoking that can contribute to overeating. For quitters, it is essential, from the start, to ensure that they do not overeat and plan an increase in activity levels to offset any increase in weight associated with cessation.[21]

Some medicines include weight gain as a side-effect.[16] The atypical antipsychotic agents – aripiprazole being the exception – can have a profound effect on the weight of patients. Many such individuals live in sheltered accommodation, and very often for supervisory reasons find it difficult, through lack of awareness, to eat a healthy diet and get sufficient exercise, while others have an entirely chaotic lifestyle and gain considerable weight while on these drugs. Furthermore, individuals with serious mental health problems often fall into a chasm between primary care, which believes that the hospital setting is inappropriate for these individuals, and secondary care, which adequately manages the mental, but not the physical aspects of the condition, which may therefore be overlooked.

A crucial aspect of the assessment and drug management of obese patients is the recognition and identification of drugs which may induce weight gain. Treatment of conditions such as diabetes and mental health disorders should always include an assessment of factors such as weight, and attempts be made to minimise exacerbations. Drugs that induce weight gain include:

- *antipsychotics*, especially olanzapine (Zyprexa). Aripiprazole (Abilify) induces the least weight gain.
- *antidepressants* including tricyclics, selective serotonin reuptake inhibitors (SSRIs), monoamine oxidase inhibitors (MAOIs) and mirtazapine (Zispin) and lithium
- *corticosteroids* may cause weight gain by fat redistribution causing truncal obesity, 'buffalo hump' and 'moon face', and also by fluid retention
- oral *contraceptive* and progesterogenic compounds
- *beta-blockers* may cause weight gain, and restrict physical activity because of fatigue
- oral *hypoglycaemics*, including glitazones and sulphonylureas, have been shown to increase weight so that the National Institute for Health and Clinical Excellence (NICE) has advised against sulphonylureas in overweight patients
- *insulin* has a direct weight gain effect, which is compounded by the risk of hypoglycaemic episodes, meaning that patients will often eat sweet food to restrict drops in blood sugar. Modern basal insulins have reduced the likelihood of weight gain
- *anticonvulsants*: weight gain has been documented with some agents (phenytoin, sodium valproate)
- *antihistamines* may cause weight gain though it is more pronounced in older agents
- *pizotifen*, used as a prophylactic migraine treatment, increases the appetite and can lead to weight gain.

Facts and figures

There are many reasons why the population of many countries are getting fatter. In the UK the number of obese people in the population is increasing rapidly. The prevalence of obesity in England as measured by BMI is 23.6% in men and 23.8% in women and in Scotland, 22.4% men and 26% women. This compares unfavourably with 1983 when the prevalence of obesity was 6% in men and 8% in women. A prediction of trends in obesity in England suggests that 26% men and 28% women will be clinically obese by 2010.[1] The latest data from the American National Centre for Health Statistics show that 30% of American adults aged 20 years of age and older – over 60 million people – are obese.[22]

Epidemiological surveys of England indicate that the prevalence of overweight and obesity in adults has trebled in the 25 years from 1980 to 2005 with almost 24 million adults being either overweight or obese in 2004. Furthermore, 0.9% of men and 2.6% of women are classified as morbidly obese with a BMI of over 40 kg/m^2.

An increase in waist circumference was also notable in 2004 with approximately 31% of men and 41% of women classified as having a raised waist circumference (>102 cm in men, >88 cm in women), demonstrating that more and more women are usurping the traditionally male 'apple' shape pattern of central obesity.

In children, the prevalence of obesity, as defined by BMI above the 95th percentile, is also rising. Figures suggest that over 16% of boys and girls aged 2–15 years were obese compared with 10% of boys and around 12% of girls in 1995. A further 14% of boys and girls were estimated to be overweight (defined as a BMI between the 85th and 95th percentiles) compared with around 13% of males and females in 1995. There are social inequalities in the prevalence of obesity in children, and children with at least one overweight or obese parent are at greater risk of obesity.

Across the UK there are differences in the prevalence of obesity. The average weight of men and women is higher in Northern Ireland compared with England and Scotland. Wales has experienced a recent surge in obesity levels. Other countries in Europe have a much lower prevalence of obesity compared with the UK, for example, in Finland just 1 in 10 women is obese compared with 1 in 5 in England.[4]

Although the average BMI in the UK has been rising in a linear fashion since the beginning of the last century, studies have identified that, particularly since the early 1980s, something has been occurring in people's lifestyle that has caused a significant shift in BMI measurement towards overweight and obesity. This phenomenon has been population-wide, not just affecting those who were already overweight or obese and getting fatter. Shifts in lifestyle trends are having a significant impact yet they are complex, subtle and difficult to tie down.

The cost of obesity

United Kingdom

In addition to its impact on health, obesity also has financial consequences for the National Health Service (NHS) and the broader UK economy with an estimated cost of at least £500 million a year in treatment costs to the NHS, and possibly in excess of £200 million to the wider economy.[14] These healthcare costs are predicted to escalate over the next few years as the number of obese people in the population increases. The economic and human cost of obesity is estimated to be very high with 1.8 million sick days a year and 30 000 deaths a year resulting in 40 000 lost years of working life. The estimated cost of obesity is £0.5 billion each year to the NHS and £2 billion each year to the wider economy.[23]

The Health Select Committee[14] reported that the cost of obesity in England is between £3.3 and £3.7 billion per year. This figure is 27–42% higher than the previous estimate by the National Audit Office[1], because of higher NHS and drug costs, the availability of more accurate data, the inclusion of co-morbidities and the increased prevalence of obesity. The HSC estimate includes £49 million for treating obesity, £1.1 billion for treating the consequences of obesity, and indirect costs of £1.1 billion for premature death and £1.45 billion for sickness absence.

Other EU states

Although British and Greek rates of obesity have risen faster than, for example, Italian or French, it appears that there is a general pan-European trend, whether Europe is defined as the 'old' European Union of 15 member states, the 'new' of 25 or the United Nations' definition of the European Region which includes 51 member states.[24]

Ireland ranks fourth in prevalence for overweight and obesity in men in the EU and seventh for women; 39% of adults in Ireland are overweight and 18% obese.[25] The in-patient cost to the Irish healthcare services in 2003 was estimated at €30 million. Indeed this was sufficiently serious to cause the Irish government to set up the National Taskforce on Obesity in 2004.

In the Netherlands, the proportion of the country's total general practitioner (family doctor) expenditure attributable to obesity and overweight has been estimated at around 3–4%.[26] In France, by 1995, obesity was already accounting for 2% of total healthcare costs[27]

United States

By 2025 it is estimated that up to 50% of the US population will be obese.[22]

Using BMI as a key indicator of the prevalence of overweight and obese individuals within the population, the increase is best seen in the US, where robust data have been available from the 1960s. The National Health and Nutrition Examination Study carried out during 1976 and 1980 showed that 52% of men and 42% in women were overweight (BMI >25 kg/m^2). When the study was repeated during the years 1988 to 1994, 60% of men and 51% of women were found to be overweight. This trend was not only occurring in those who were overweight but was occurring across the population, indicating a lifestyle rather than a genetic cause.

Yet the impact of obesity is not the same for each ethnic group. In women, 82% of non-Hispanic blacks are overweight, compared with 75% of Mexican Americans and 58% of non-Hispanic white women. Seventy-six percent of Mexican American men are overweight, compared with 71% of non-Hispanic white men and 69% of non-Hispanic black men.

Family income influences obesity. Women with lower income have a 50% higher risk of developing obesity than those with higher income. The reason is thought to be the preferential purchasing of high-fat, high-carbohydrate foods, which may be less expensive than healthy foods such as fruit and vegetables.

The burden of obesity is becoming clearer. One study suggests that 40-year-old female nonsmokers lost 3.3 years from their lifespan, and 40-year-old male nonsmokers lost 3.1 years of life expectancy because of being overweight. The same groups lost 7.1 years and 5.8 years respectively because of obesity. Add obesity to smoking, the other major public health issue, and the impact on mortality is dramatic. Obese female smokers lose 13.3 years of life expectancy and obese male smokers lose 13.7 years – the years of life lost are doubled.[6]

Rest of the world

The World Health Organization predicts that globally in 2005 1.6 billion adults were overweight and of these 400 million adults were classified obese.[4] There is no region anywhere in the world that has no obesity problem; levels range from below 5% in China, Japan and certain African nations, to over 75% in urban Samoa. Surprisingly the trends are more pronounced in developing countries where there is a sudden increase in wealth – clearly a rapid increase in the standard of living has a negative impact on public health.

In developing countries, the increase in obesity has been even more rapid than in developed countries. In Mauritius, for example, from 1987 to 1992 the prevalence of people overweight increased by 10%. In Kuwait the prevalence of obesity at the beginning of the 1990s was a high as 32% in men and 41% in women.

Communities that exhibit high levels of obesity and the highest prevalence of type 2 diabetes are often wealthy and geographically isolated, such as the island communities of Malta and in Polynesia. These nations are often incapable of producing their own food because of water or soil restrictions. Currently, in Europe, Malta has the highest levels of obesity in children with over 50% of 10 year olds with a BMI indicating they are overweight.[4] Because of their wealth, they are capable of importing high-energy foods that become the staple diet of the population, particularly the young. The foods need to have a long shelf life and to be easily transported, and are culturally prized, particularly where education levels are low. Coupled with this are the physical inactivity that accompanies increased wealth, and a hot climate that does not support much exercise, and it is easy to see why obesity levels rise so dramatically.

Conclusion

The future

The Foresight Report[28] published in November 2007 took a long-term (40-year) view of obesity in the UK. It was created by a group of experts in the field of obesity and nutrition and it set out the projections for obesity and its impact on public health as well as the cost to the NHS. It concluded that the problem of obesity in the population could cost the UK an additional £45 billion and take 30 years to turn around. It predicted that 60% of men and 50% of women and 25% of children will be obese by 2050.

The report accepts the fact that humans, because of their biology, are predisposed to become fat but that, in the past, this only happened to a few in the population. Yet, since the 1970s, because of cultural, environmental and social changes, the UK has witnessed the emergence of an 'obesogenic' environment and as a result, across the population, people have been becoming fatter. This they term 'passive obesity'.

The report accepts that policies aimed at individuals and small-scale local interventions are unlikely to be successful. What is called for is effective action toward prevention at a population level. There is a call for the production and promotion of healthy diets, a redesign of the built environment with more promotion of walking and for a cultural change to shift societal views on food and activity.

Interestingly the report compares the necessary action on obesity with the necessary action on climate change, suggesting that both problems will require considerable societal attitudinal change and cross-government action. It goes on to say that tackling both issues together could bring benefits to both. For example, with more walking and cycling and a built environment to support this, there would less traffic congestion as well as a healthier population.

References

1. National Audit Office. *Tackling Obesity in England*. London: The Stationary Office, 2001.
2. Egger G, Swinburn B. An 'ecological' approach to the obesity pandemic. *BMJ* 1997; 315: 477–480.
3. Royal College of Physicians. *Anti-obesity drugs – Guidance on appropriate prescribing and management: A report of a working party of the Nutrition Committee of the Royal College of Physicians*. London: Royal College of Physicians, 2003.
4. WHO *Global strategy on diet, physical activity and health*. Geneva: World Health Assembly, 2004.
5. Johnson A (UK Secretary of State for Health) Reported in *Independent on Sunday*, 14 Oct 2007.
6. Smith-Maguire J. *Fit for Consumption: sociology and the business of fitness*. Amazon Books, 2008.
7. Wanless D. *Securing Our Future Health: taking a long-term view*. London: HM Treasury, 2002.
8. Waine C. Personal communication. MHRA annual conference, Birmingham, 2007.
9. Wanless D. *Securing Good Health for the Whole Population*. London: HM Treasury, 2004.
10. World Health Organization. *World Health Report 2002*. Geneva: WHO, 2002.
11. Stearns P. *Fat History: bodies and beauty in the modern West*, New York: New York University Press, 1997.
12. World Health Organization/Food & Agricultural Organization. *Diet, Nutrition and the Prevention of Chronic Diseases*. WHO Technical Report Series 916. Geneva: WHO/FAO, 2003.
13. Cannon G, Einzig H. *Dieting Makes You Fat*. London: Sphere, 1983.
14. House of Commons Health Committee. *Obesity*. London: The Stationery Office, 2004.
15. Schlosser E. *Fast Food Nation*. London: Penguin Books, 2002.
16. Waine C. *Obesity and Weight Management in Primary Care*. Oxford: Blackwell, 2002.
17. Bolton-Smith C, Woodward M. Dietary composition and fat to sugar ratios in relation to obesity. *Int J Obes* 1994; 18: 820–828.
18. Burke J *et al*. Correlates of obesity in young black and white women: the CARDIA Study. *Am J Public Health* 1992; 82: 1621–1625.
19. Colhoun H, Prescott-Clarke P, eds. *Health Survey for England 1994: a survey carried out on behalf of DoH*, vol. 1. London: HMSO, 1996.
20. Van Gaal L. *Managing Obesity and Diabetes*. London: Science Press, 2003.
21. Maguire T, *et al*. A randomized controlled trial of a smoking cessation intervention based in community pharmacies. *Addiction* 2001; 96: 325–331.
22. US Surgeon General. *A Call to Action to Prevent and Decrease Overweight and Obesity 2001*. Rockville, MD: US Department of Health and Human Services, Public Health Service, Office of the Surgeon General, 2001.
23. Costain L. *Diet Trials: how to succeed at dieting*. London: BBC Worldwide, 2003.
24. Lang T *et al*. *Intersectoral Food and Nutrition Policy Development: a manual for decision-makers*. Copenhagen: World Health Organization, 2001.
25. O'Shea D. The obesity epidemic – pharmacists can make a difference. *Irish Pharm* 2006; 8: 26–28.
26. Kemper H C *et al*. The prevention and treatment of overweight and obesity. Summary of the advisory report by the Health Council of The Netherlands. *Neth J Med* 2004; 62: 10–71.
27. Levy E *et al*. The economic cost of obesity: the French situation, *Int J Obes Relat Metab Disord* 1995; 19: 788–792.
28. King M *et al*. *Foresight Project Report. Tackling Obesities: future choices*. London: Government Office For Science, 2007.

2

Defining the problem

Chapter 1 discussed the scale of the obesity problem using current epidemiological data. What is clear from this extensive body of data is that in the past 30 years there has been an alarming increase in the numbers of people in the populations of developed nations who are either overweight or obese. There are also robust data (considered in Chapter 3) causally linking increased body weight with increased morbidity and higher mortality rates. Based on this data there is, understandably, a necessity from a public health perspective for something to be done, specifically to reduce the potential health burden that obesity will create in coming years. This chapter considers the definitions of obesity and the measures employed to define the problem and, more importantly perhaps, to show how effective these measures are in practice.

An 'ideal' measure of obesity would be one that is accurate, precise, and simple to perform. In addition it would be inexpensive, non-invasive and would be correlated directly with disease risk. Disease risk correlation should also work in reverse, i.e. a reduction in this ideal measure would be associated with a quantifiable reduction in disease risk both in individuals and in a population.

An ideal objective measure of obesity is yet to be found. In its absence there is a reliance on the use of a number of measures, each assessing a different aspect of obesity, for example, weight, body mass index (BMI) and total and regional adiposity; each of these measure will have limitations that must be taken into account when assessing the clinical significance of the measure. Yet when used together a number of these measures can provide a good estimate of absolute disease risk. The problem, as stated in Chapter 1, is that obesity is a state and only one of a number of independent risk factor for disease, rather than being a disease in itself. What is clear is that the more clinical measures used, the better the estimate of disease risk in a specific individual or a population. For example, metabolic syndrome, a condition in which obesity is a key element, will require that other measures are used as well, for example, blood glucose concentration, blood pressure measurement and serum cholesterol, to identify specific patients at increased risk and for whom interventions can be initiated.

Weight

Body weight in kilograms is the simplest of anthropometric measures to undertake and using an appropriate set of scales is perhaps the easiest and most accessible measure available to practitioners. But bathroom scales have been a feature of British and American homes for over 40 years yet there is little to suggest their ubiquity has contributed to a reduction in national waistlines.

Whereas a simple measure of body mass in terms of weight (kg) is of little predictive value for disease risk, it does provide a basis for the calculation of BMI that is better at assessing disease risk. Weight measurement will allow us to consider two features of a clinical assessment: accuracy and precision, that are critical to the usefulness of the measure (or test result) in predicting clinical consequences.

Accuracy is an estimate of how well a test result gives the right answer – hits the metaphorical bull's eye (figure 2.1). Accuracy of any clinical test is dependent on a number of factors, including the ability of the individual or technician to undertake the measure; this will include the training they received and the quality of the equipment used.

Precision is the ability of the testing system, i.e. the same set of scales to give the same result each time the measure is taken. To weigh yourself 10 times on your bathroom scales over a 10-minute period is unlikely to show, within the 10 weights recorded, much variation. A testing system that gives very little variation between test results of repeated tests is said to be precise (see figure 2.1). Precision therefore is getting the right answer and getting it every time. Precision will vary from testing system to testing system and will be dependent on the processes used. Some clinical tests, even those using

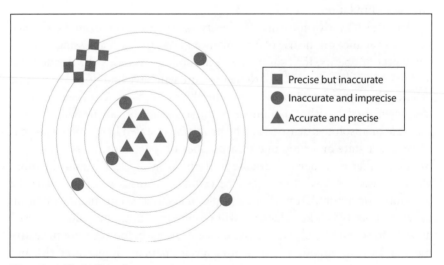

Figure 2.1 The 'bull's eye'.

good quality equipment, can produce acceptable variations in results of up to 10% in a series of tests, for example, serum cholesterol evaluation. So a test must be accurate – give the right result – and it must be precise – give that result each time.

Using a set of weighing scales is relatively easy for most to do and would not require much specialist training. However the quality of the equipment can vary. It is unlikely that the standard bathroom scales – even when a perfect match for the Italian marble tiles – is unlikely to be acceptable to an inspector from 'weights and measures', and where the scales are to be used to monitor a patient's health closely. Indeed someone who decides to weigh her or himself on a range of scales – at home, at work and in the local pharmacy, for example, is likely to get range of results and this will compromise precision.

Quality control of testing systems

Quality, and the application of a quality mark to a piece of equipment, is key to ensuring that weighing scales are standardised and are therefore accurate within a small defined margin. Using such equipment will ensure that an accurate measure is gained. Calibration of the equipment will be necessary on a regular basis as part of the quality control of the equipment but stamped equipment has legal restrictions about re-calibration.

In general, two classes of weighing equipment are used in clinical practice: class III (more sensitive, small divisions) and class IV (less sensitive, large divisions). Whereas class III equipment is preferable to class IV, which includes domestic scales, it can be used for recording patients' weight

---

Box 2.1 *Weights and measures tips provided by Local Authorities Coordinators of Regulatory Services (LACORS)*

- A system for regularly checking the accuracy of weighing equipment should be in place, and adjustments should be made if errors are noted.
- The quality of equipment should be considered before purchasing.
- Staff using the equipment should be trained appropriately.
- All medical equipment bought after 1 Jan 2003 and used for weighing patients 'for the purpose of monitoring, diagnosis and medical treatment' should be verified, stamped or stickered.
- Where measurements can be taken in metric and imperial units, care must be exercised as errors can occur where staff mis-read pounds for kilograms.

and calculating BMI. Baby-weighers need to be more accurate as they are used to calculate medicine dosages and therefore must be class III.

In the UK, weighing equipment must meet legal standards, and LACORS (Local Authorities Coordinators of Regulatory Services), on behalf of local authority trading standards departments, offer their services to health trusts to ensure that weighting equipment is accurate (box 2.1). Inspectors will not routinely visit general practitioner surgeries or pharmacies but are happy to visit on request by contacting the local trading standard department.

Clinical testing systems, be they serum cholesterol results produced by a certified laboratory using costly equipment or a simple weight measurement undertaken by individuals on their bathroom scales need to be both accurate (giving the true result) and precise (giving the result each time a measure is made). Only when clinical tests are accurate and precise do they become meaningful in terms of producing epidemiological evidence for a link with disease risk within a population.

Body mass index

Accuracy and precision aside, a simple body weight measurement (mass) is poorly linked to disease risk irrespective of how accurate and precise the measure is. Tall people with the same degree of adiposity as a small person will have no greater risk of coronary heart disease (CHD) or of developing type 2 diabetes but will be heavier. For this reason body mass index is the anthropometric measure used in most epidemiological studies.

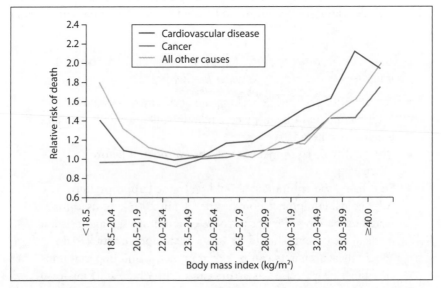

Figure 2.2 High BMI increases the risk of mortality in women. © (1999) Massachusetts Medical Society. All rights reserved.

Use this chart to work out the health risk attached to your own body shape. It is suitable for both men and women and children over 5 yrs.

The size of your waist circumference is a good indicator of your overall health risk. Why is this?

Excess fat which is found deep down in the region of the stomach gives someone a large waist circumference and an 'apple' shape. This is often associated with risk factors for serious conditions such as heart disease, raised blood pressure, diabetes and some types of cancer.

Excess fat which is found under the skin, around the bottom, hips and thighs gives someone a smaller waist circumference and a 'pear' shape. This is generally accepted to be less harmful to health.

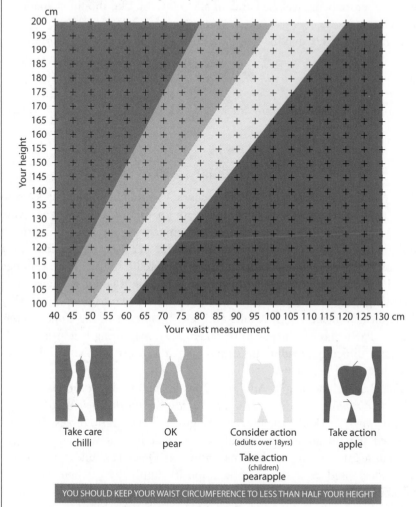

Take care
chilli

OK
pear

Consider action
(adults over 18yrs)
Take action
(children)
pearapple

Take action
apple

YOU SHOULD KEEP YOUR WAIST CIRCUMFERENCE TO LESS THAN HALF YOUR HEIGHT

• Matching your height to your smallest waist circumference, where does your shape fall in the chart?

• If your shape is in the 'chilli' region, you should Take Care. You will not need to decrease your waistline.

• If your shape is in the 'pear' region, you have a healthy OK shape.

• If your shape falls in the 'pearapple' region (particularly the upper end), you should Consider Action (adults over 18yrs) or Take Action (children over 5 yrs). Make certain that you don't increase your waistline any more.

• If your shape falls in the 'apple' region, your health is probably at risk. Why not talk to your GP and Take Action?

Figure 2.3   The Ashwell Shape Chart. © Dr Margaret Ashwell OBE. Reproduced with permission.

BMI has been identified as an independent risk factor for the development of CHD[2] specifically in all-cause mortality and it holds true when consideration is taken of other risks, such as smoking (figures 2.2 and 2.3). It requires a relatively simple measure of height and weight. Height can be measured by a suitably installed stadiometer. Clients should remove their shoes before the measure is undertaken. Clients should remove all outdoor clothing before being weighed and an allowance of 1 kg should be made for light clothing.

Body mass index may be calculated using the following equation:

$$\text{BMI} = \frac{\text{weight (kg)}}{\text{height (m}^2)}$$

An example is given below for a male who weighs 75 kg and is 1.72 m tall.

$$\text{BMI} = \frac{75 \text{ kg}}{(1.72 \text{ m})^2} = \frac{75}{2.95} = 25.4$$

Clearly, in the calculation of BMI, the accuracy of weight and height is essential – particularly height – since any error in this measurement is being squared and therefore will have a greater impact on the final measure. In addition, precision becomes important when further measures are made, for example, following an intervention that is expected to bring about a change in BMI. If the test is poorly performed and precision is not managed then any change, or lack of change, in BMI, could be down to the poor quality of the measurement of test results and not the impact of the clinical intervention. Particular care needs to be taken when measuring height in people who have difficulty standing up straight, such as those with spinal or other musculoskeletal problems.

The Belgian sociologist Adolphe Quetelet published *Recherches sur le poids de l'homme aux différent âges* (*Researches on the weights of man at different ages*) in 1833 – the first ever height-to-weight ratio tables. Quetelet observed that in adults of normal size, weight is proportional to height squared, a calculation that became known as Quetelet's index, and which was widely used as a measure of adiposity until 1972, when Keys and colleagues proposed its re-invention as the body mass index used today.[3]

BMI is a crude measure of obesity. The risk to health associated with BMI categories is shown in table 2.1, yet even though this is a widely used measure of obesity, BMI is only a crude predictor of disease risk in an individual. BMI does not discriminate between muscle mass (lean tissue) and adipose tissue (fatness). For example, someone who starts an exercise programme and as a result achieves a reduction in adipose tissue but an increase in muscle mass, associated with an increase in fibrous and vascular tissue, will not show a reduction in BMI. All these non-fat tissues have a

Table 2.1 BMI, obesity and health risk		
BMI	Category	Risk to health
<20	Underweight	Moderate
20–25	Optimal weight	None
25–30	Overweight	Moderate
30–39	Obese	Significant
≥40	Grossly obese	Highly significant

higher density (1.0 g/mL) compared with fat (0.7 g/mL) and results in a reduction in disease risk but is not be accompanied by a reduction in BMI.

Some population groups, such as Asians and older people, have co-morbidity risk factors that would not fit with the risk categories given in table 2.1. An Asian adult's risk is greater at lower BMI and older people have less risk at higher BMI. There is some controversy in recent years over the value of a BMI measurement in the management of obesity. Clearly, when the front row of the Irish rugby team would all be classed as obese, there are some questions to be asked about the general validity of this measure. The simple answer is that the usefulness of a BMI measure, as a measure of disease risk, is down to an individual's daily activity levels. Where a patient has a sedentary lifestyle there is a stronger correlation with BMI and disease risk than where the patient is very active, such as an international rugby player.

BMI and children

With the alarming rise in childhood obesity in recent years, and the consequences that this implies regarding public health in future years, the usefulness of BMI in children has been considered in detail. Clearly children should put on weight over the years of growth – this is natural – and it is only excess weight gain, fatness, that presents a problem. No absolute BMI standards exist to classify children and adolescents as overweight or obese. Expert panels recommend BMI-for-age to identify the increasing number of children and adolescents at the upper end of the distribution who are either overweight (those children at or above the 95th percentile) or at risk of being overweight (those at or above the 85th percentile but below the 95th percentile).[4] The Child Growth Foundation in the UK supplies the Cole calculator that enables the height and weight for boys and girls to be used not only to calculate the current BMI, but also to relate this to the adult BMI. Charts have been provided for girls and boys for ages birth to 20 years (figures 2.4 and 2.5), which allow comparison of a child at a certain age

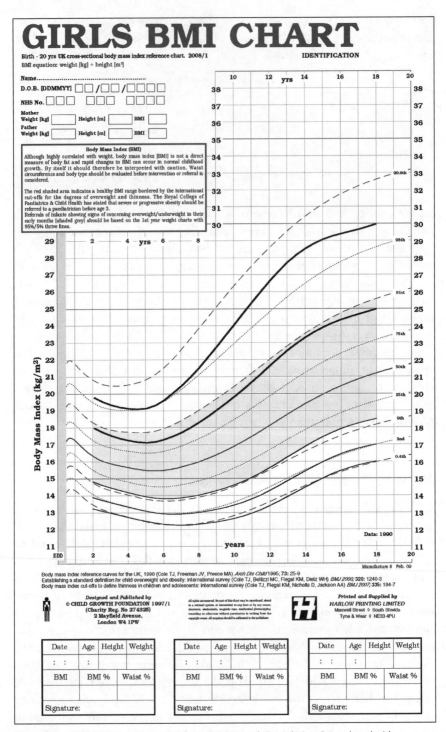

Figure 2.4 Girls' BMI chart. Courtesy of the Child Growth Foundation. Reproduced with permission.

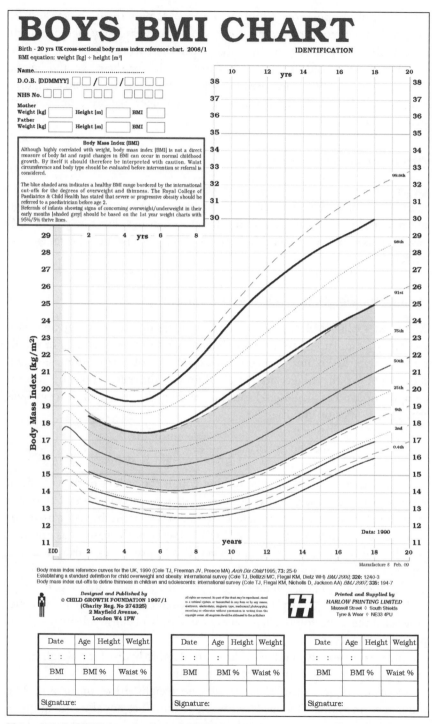

Figure 2.5 Boys' BMI chart. Courtesy of the Child Growth Foundation. Reproduced with permission.

with the child population. Children whose BMI puts them above the 98th percentile are of concern, as this group would be regarded as obese and will potentially need expert help and advice. Children whose BMI is above the 91st percentile would be regarded as overweight for their age and height. These charts are a good measure of the risk of adult obesity, as those children with a second rise in weight occurring at a younger age are more likely to become obese adults.

Other measures of adiposity

Other measures of obesity, such as the bioelectrical impedance test and immersion tests, are more accurate and precise in predicting disease risk but not practical in the primary care or pharmacy settings. For this reason BMI is widely used and is a useful indicator of risk in someone who takes little exercise.

Hydrostatic weighing: Archimedes' principle

Archimedes (287–212 BC) discovered that water displacement by an object is directly proportional to its mass: the famous 'Eureka!' moment. In simple terms, where the volume of water displaced by an object on immersion and the weight of the object in air are known, the percentage of specific component can be calculated. From this Archimedes reasoned the principles that give us specific gravity:

$$\text{specific gravity} = \frac{\text{weight in air}}{\text{loss of weight in water}}$$

An object looses weight in water that equals the weight of the volume of water it displaces. The object's specific gravity refers to the mass of an object in air divided by its loss of weight in water. Whereas Archimedes used this to estimate and to prove that King Hieron of Syracuse's crown was not pure gold but an amalgam of gold and silver, this approach can also be use to determine a body's volume. Dividing body mass by its volume yields body density (density = mass/volume) and from this, an estimate of percentage body fat. Specific gravity is an object's heaviness related to its volume. Objects of the same volume may vary considerably in density defined as mass per unit volume.

There is now considerable evidence to support hydrostatic weighting as an accurate estimate of the body's fat content.

As an example, consider a person who weighs 50 kg in air and 2 kg submerged in water. The displaced water is therefore equal to 48 kg or 48 litres (48 000 cm^3). It is important to appreciate that the temperature of the water is critical in this assessment.

$$\text{density} = \frac{50\,000}{48\,000} = 1.0417 \text{ g/cm}^2$$

The density of fat tissue is taken as 0.90 g/cm³ and the density of fat-free tissue (bone and muscle) is 1.10 g/cm³.

The Siri equation is one of a number of equations used to calculate body mass and is based on the fact that body fat density and non-fat density remains relatively constant among individuals, despite large individual variations in total fat and non-fat (bone and tissue). This equation is given as:

$$\text{percentage body fat} = \frac{495}{\text{body density}} - 450.$$

Taking our example above:

$$\text{percentage body fat} = \frac{495}{1.0417} - 450 = 25.2\%.$$

Subcutaneous fat measurement

The rationale for using skinfold to estimate body fat comes from the inter-relationships among three factors:

- adipose tissue directly beneath the skin (subcutaneous fat)
- internal fat
- whole-body density.

As far back as the 1930s, a calliper was used to accurately measure subcutaneous fat at selected anatomic sites. Measuring skinfold thickness requires firmly grasping a fold of skin and subcutaneous fat with thumb and forefingers, pulling it away from the underlying muscle tissue. When calibrated the pincers should exert a constant tension of 10 g/mm at the point of contact on the two layers of skin plus its subcutaneous fat when recorded within two seconds after applying the full force of the calliper.

Successful measurement of subcutaneous fat by this method, although it appears simple, requires considerable experience on behalf of the technician. Careful attention to detail usually ensures a high measurement reproducibility.

Common sites for skinfold measurements include: triceps, subscapular, suprailiac, abdominal and upper thigh sites. Two or three measurements in rotational order at each site with the subject standing are recommended. The average value represents the skinfold score.

Skinfold measurements, while largely not used in UK clinical practice, provide meaningful information about body fat and its distribution. The measurement is not used more widely because of the need for competence

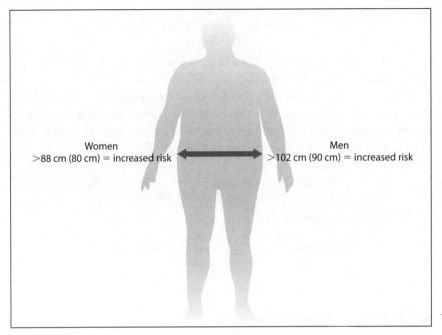

Women
>88 cm (80 cm) = increased risk

Men
>102 cm (90 cm) = increased risk

Figure 2.6 Body fat distribution: apple-shaped obesity.

in the proper use of the technique. In extremely obese people, the skinfold thickness often exceeds the width of the calliper's jaws. The quality of the skinfold calliper used can also contribute to errors.[5]

Central obesity

Where fatness or increased amounts of adipose tissue exist on the body this is linked to the degree of disease risk. For example, central obesity, common in males, indicates a greater risk of developing CHD and type 2 diabetes. This central obesity is known as the 'apple' shape and contrasts with the 'pear' shape, more common in females, where the obesity occurs on the hips and increases the risk of osteoarthritic disease (figure 2.6).

An increase in fat deposition around the abdomen – the apple shape – is the main risk factor, rather than obesity itself, for the development of type 2 diabetes. Adipose tissue in the abdominal cavity has a high lipolytic rate that releases free fatty acids that drain directly into the liver via the portal circulation. Flooding of the liver in this manner has a direct impact on hepatic glucose homeostasis: insulin-mediated inhibition of gluconeogenesis is reduced and peripheral muscle uptake of glucose is impaired. Insulin resistance develops and impaired glucose tolerance results in hyper-insulinaemia and profound dyslipidaemias. With impaired clearance there

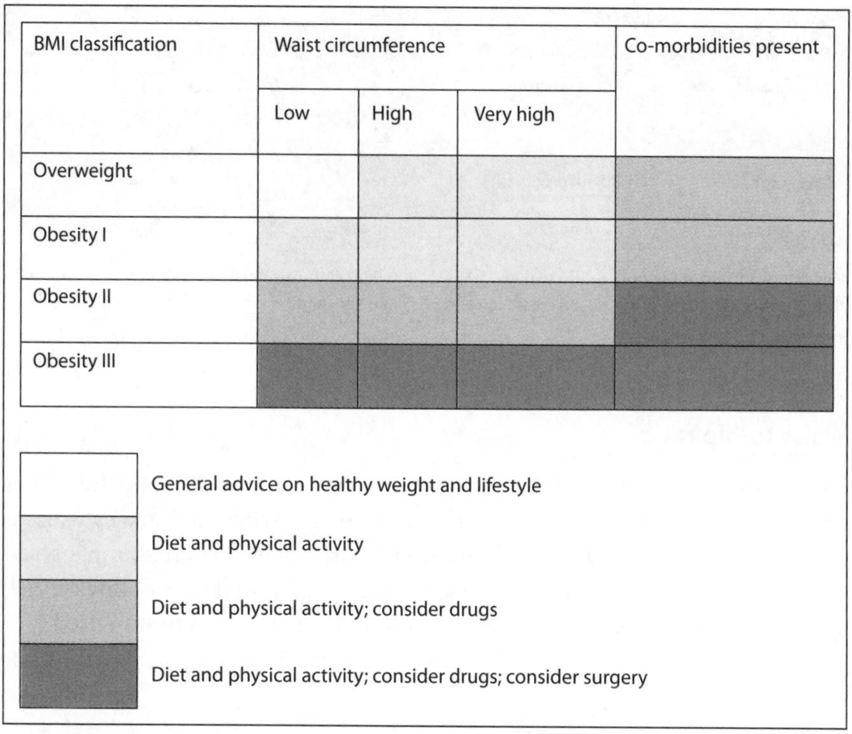

BMI classification	Waist circumference			Co-morbidities present
	Low	High	Very high	
Overweight				
Obesity I				
Obesity II				
Obesity III				

General advice on healthy weight and lifestyle

Diet and physical activity

Diet and physical activity; consider drugs

Diet and physical activity; consider drugs; consider surgery

Figure 2.7 Levels of intervention. Reproduced from Lean *et al.*[6]

are raised plasma triglycerides, reduced high-density lipoprotein (HDL) cholesterol, which are cardioprotective, and high levels of low-density lipoprotein (LDL) cholesterol, which generate the small, atherogenic LDL particles that contribute directly to coronary heart disease.

Therefore BMI, in conjunction with a waist circumference, provides a better measure of disease risk[6] (tables 2.2 and 2.3).

Figure 2.7 shows levels of interventions.[6]

Table 2.2 BMI classifications

Classification	BMI (kg/m²)
Healthy weight	18.5–24.9
Overweight	25–29.9
Obesity I	30–34.9
Obesity II	35–39.9
Obesity III	≥40

Table 2.3 Disease risk in relation to BMI and waist circumference

BMI classification	Waist circumference*		
	Low	High	Very high
Overweight	No increased risk	Increased risk	High risk
Obesity I	Increased risk	High risk	Very high risk

*For men, waist circumference of <94 cm is low, 94–102 cm is high and >102 cm is very high; for women, waist circumference of <80 cm is low, 80–88 cm is high and >88 cm is very high.

Waist-to-hip ratio

The waist-to-hip ratio for a female should be less than 0.9 and for males should be less than 0.8. There is an increased risk where a female's waist is greater than 88 cm and a male's waist is greater than 102 cm. Simple waist circumference measurement (figure 2.8) is as good a predictor of disease risk as waist-to-hip ratio, however, and so the latter is less commonly used.[7]

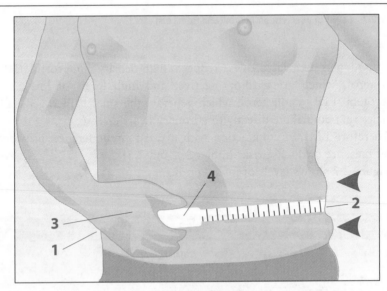

(1) Place a tape measure around the bare abdomen just above the hip bone.
(2) Position the tape measure parallel to the floor, midway between the top of the the iliac crest and the lower rib margin on each side.
(3) Ensure the tape measure is snug, but not compressed against the skin.
(4) As the individual relaxes and exhales, the waist measurement can be taken.

Figure 2.8 Guide to measuring waist circumference.

Table 2.4 Disease risk and waist circumference in white men		
Risk	Men (cm)	Women (cm)
Low	<94	<80
Increased	>94–101.9	>80–87.9
High	≥102	≥88

Waist circumference

Waist circumference is at least as good an indicator of total body fat as BMI and is also the best predictor of visceral fat (table 2.4).

Waist measurement is best undertaken using a specially designed tape measure. Patients should be asked not to hold their stomach in and a constant-tension, spring-loaded tape device reduces errors from overtightening. The tape should be placed around the abdomen across the soft tissue between the lower rib margin and iliac crest (right and left protrusions of the pelvic bone) and measurement made horizontally at the end of gentle expiration. In very obese subjects and those who have lost considerable weight, the measurement is not reliable because of sagging waist circumference at the umbilicus. For this reason a change in body fat may not be detected by waist circumference measurement in very fat people when the abdominal mass is pendulous.[8]

Computer tomography

Computed tomography (CT) generates detailed cross-sectional, two-dimensional radiographic images of body segments when an X-ray beam passes through tissues of different densities. The CT scan produces pictorial and quantitative information about total tissue area, total fat and muscle area, and thickness and volume of tissues within an organ. Indeed, studies have demonstrated the efficacy of CT scans to establish the relationship between simple anthropometric measures (skinfolds and waist girth) at the abdomen and total abdominal fat volume measured from single or multiple pictorial 'slices' through this region. This technique suggests a strong association between waist circumference and deep visceral adipose tissue. It is deep abdominal adipose tissue that has the best causal relationship between fat and risk of type 2 diabetes, hypertension and cardiovascular disease.[9] The increased visceral fat simply squeezes the internal organs greatly increasing disease risk.

Magnetic resonance imaging

Magnetic resonance imaging (MRI) provides an invaluable, non-invasive assessment of the body's tissue compartments. Computer software can subtract fat and bony tissues given the different densities of these tissues.

Whereas both CT and MRI are very precise measures of body fat, and as a consequence obesity, they need expensive equipment that requires highly competent operators, which is not practical in the clinic or in the pharmacy.

Other clinical tests

Although blood pressure, blood glucose concentration and serum cholesterol determination do not measure directly body fatness or obesity, they are relevant in the community pharmacy and primary care setting since they are relevant to the risk posed by obesity including development of hypertension, cardiovascular disease and type 2 diabetes.

Blood pressure

A raised blood pressure is a major risk factor in the development of coronary heart disease and is a key component of metabolic syndrome. Both raised diastolic and systolic pressure have been implicated and there is much debate as to which is more important.

Blood pressure varies during each beat of the heart (cardiac cycle). The contraction of the ventricles (systole) sends a pressure wave radiating down the major arteries and the pressure produced is referred to as the systolic blood pressure. When the ventricles are filling with blood (dystole) the pressure in the arteries is reduced to the lowest level and this is termed diastolic blood pressure.

Conventionally blood pressure is measured in the brachial artery at a point just above the elbow. When an external pressure is applied to the upper arm such as by inflating a cuff, as the pressure increases blood flow through the artery becomes more restricted until a pressure is reached where the cuff pressure exceeds the highest pressure (systolic) in the artery. At this point all blood flow into the arm ceases.

If the cuff is then deflated to a pressure at which the systolic pressure just exceeds the cuff pressure, blood will be forced through the artery at this point in the heart beat. Since the pressure in the artery will very quickly drop towards the diastolic pressure, it will snap closed as the cuff pressure again exceeds the artery pressure. This artery closing produces a sound, the Korotkoff sound. When the Korotkoff sound first appears, the pressure observed represents the systolic pressure. Diastolic pressure is the measurement recorded when the Korotkoff sounds become 'muffled' (phase IV) or disappears (phase V). The custom in the UK is to measure phase 1V blood pressure. Phase V pressure is about 5 mmHg lower. Most of the automated systems (such as those available in pharmacies), because of the technique they employ, use phase V measurements. This has the potential to confuse patients if measurements are taken in the pharmacy.

Since many factors can cause variation in blood pressure, measurement must be standardised to ensure accurate and precise results.

The quality of instrument is vitally important and it is the user's responsibility to ensure that manufactures provide appropriate quality assurance.[10] The Royal Pharmaceutical Society of Great Britain recommends that pharmacists use a semi-automatic sphygmomanometer that is accurate, robust, simple to operate and easy to clean and maintain. Pharmacists have a responsibility to maintain equipment and to have accuracy confirmed at least once yearly.

The client must be seated for at least 10 minutes before a measurement, and his/her arm supported at heart height on a bench or table. Blood pressure measured when the client is in the seated position will differ from blood pressure measured when the client is lying down. 'White-coat syndrome' should be avoided. This refers to the anxiety felt by individuals when they are having a blood pressure test in stressful surroundings, such as a doctor's surgery. The reading should be taken in a room that has a pleasant temperature; extremes of temperature will affect the result.

The size of the cuff should be matched to the size of the arm and the girth of the limb should be 2–3 times the cuff width. Ideally there should be three cuff sizes to choose from: a small cuff covering 9 cm length of artery and a standard cuff that covers 12 cm of artery, used mainly for non-obese adults. For adults who are obese and the girth of the arm exceeds 36 cm, a large size cuff should be used. A cuff that is too small will overestimate the blood pressure causing 'cuff hypertension'.

Pulse rate

Pulse rate (heart rate) is simple to measure; it only requires detection of the pulse (usually at the wrist) and a clock with a second hand. With the facing palm upright the pulse is easily located just above the wrist by simple application of the tips of the fingers and then pressing down until the pulse is detected. Pulse rate is an independent risk factor for cardiovascular disease and mortality; a raised heart rate is associated with other CHD risk factors including hypertension, dyslipidaemia, raised blood glucose and hyper-insulinaemia and being overweight and obese.[11]

Pulse rate is under both hormonal and neural control. Hormones such as adrenaline will affect heart rate but it is affected more by both the sympathetic and parasympathetic nervous system. The intrinsic activity of the sinoatrial node produces a resting heart rate of between 100 and 120 beats per minute (bpm). Parasympathetic activity dominates slowing resting heart rate, in normal health subjects, to between 55 and 70 bpm.

The benefits of pulse rate is possibly best applied as a measure of fitness. A discussion of resting pulse rate, exercise pulse rate and recovery pulse rate is given in Chapter 9 where exercise is discussed.

Blood glucose and serum cholesterol

Self-testing of both blood glucose and serum cholesterol is now possible from handheld instruments. These instruments are highly accurate and precise and quality control is normally built into the systems by the manufacturer reducing the need for elaborate quality control procedures. These tests are useful in combination with BMI and BP in overall vascular assessment of patients when providing clinical interventions.

Basal metabolic rate

Everyone requires a minimal level of energy to sustain vital functions – the basal metabolic rate (BMR). Measuring oxygen consumption under stringent conditions indirectly determines the BMR. The individual must not have eaten for 12 hours since metabolism and absorption increases energy expenditure. The individual must have total rest for 2 hours before the test and remain supine for a minimum of 30 minutes in a room that is at body temperature.

Knowledge of BMR establishes the baseline for constructing a sound programme of weight control through food restriction or regular exercise or both.

The Harris Benedict equation is a formula that uses BMR and then applies an activity factor to determine an individual's total daily energy expenditure (calories). The only factor omitted by the Harris Benedict equation is lean body mass. Leaner bodies need more calories than less lean ones, therefore this equation will be very accurate in all but the very muscular (in whom it will underestimate energy needs) and the very fat (in whom it will overestimate energy needs).[12] A detailed discussion of the Harris Benedict equation is beyond the scope of this book. It is a technically challenging equation to use and normally is used only in specialist clinical units.

A person's energy requirements can be calculated using the modified Harris Benedict equation, in which BMR is multiplied by an activity factor. BMR is calculated using the following equation:

male = 66 + (13.7 × weight in kg) + (5 × height in cm) − (6.8 × age)
female = 655 + (9.6 × weight in kg) + (1.8 × height in cm) − (4.7 × age)

and is then multiplied by a physical activity factor:

sedentary = BMR × 1.2
light activity (light exercise/sports 1–3 days/week) = BMR × 1.375
moderate activity (moderate exercise/sports 3–5 days/week) = BMR × 1.55
vigorous activity (hard exercise/sports 6–7 days a week) = BMR × 1.725
extreme activity (very hard exercise/sports and physical job) = BMR × 1.9.

This gives the number of calories a person requires, and from which 500–600 kcal daily can then be subtracted.

Conclusion

Obesity is a highly visible public health issue and is normally defined in the primary care setting using the BMI calculation. However, this simple measure has a number of drawbacks in clinical practice and is now normally used in conjunction with waist measurement to give a better estimate of disease risk in a specific individual. Other clinical measures – blood pressure, blood glucose concentration and serum cholesterol – help define metabolic syndrome and arguably give improved precision in the estimation of individual disease risk. More precise measures of obesity can be obtained using more sophisticated measures and these may give a more accurate prediction of the disease risk associated with obesity but these are not practical in the primary care setting.

References

1. Department of Health, Estates and Facilities Division Quarterly Briefing (V16.N2), 2008.
2. Calle E E *et al*. Body-mass index and mortality in a prospective cohort of US adults. *N Engl J Med* 1999; 341: 1097–1105.
3. Keys A *et al*. Indices of relative weight and obesity. *J Chron Dis* 1972; 25: 329–343.
4. Kuczmarski R *et al*. CDC growth charts, US. Advance data no 314. In: *Vital and Health Statistics*. Washington DC: Centers for Disease Control and Prevention, 2000.
5. Nindl B *et al*. Comparison of body composition assessments among lean black and white male collegiate athletes. *Med Sci Sports Exerc* 1998; 30: 769–776.
6. Lean M *et al*. Impairment of health and quality of life in people with large waist circumferences. *Lancet* 1998; 351: 853–856.
7. National Institute for Health and Clinical Excellence. *Obesity: the prevention, identification, assessment and management of overweight and obesity in adults and children*. London: NICE, 2007.
8. Wei M *et al*. Waist circumference as the best predictor of NIDDM compared to body mass index, waist/hip ratio and other anthropometric measurements in Mexican Americans – a 7 year prospective study. *Obes Res* 1997; 5: 16–23.

9. Mitsiopoulos N *et al.* Cadaver validation of skeletal muscle measurement by magnetic resonance imaging and computerized tomography. *J Appl Physiol* 1998; 85: 115–122.

10. Royal Pharmaceutical Society of Great Britain. *Practice Guidance on Testing Body Fluids*. London: RPSGB, 2003.

11. Cook S *et al.* High heart rate: a cardiovascular risk factor? *Eur Heart J* 2006; 27: 2387–2393.

12. Starling R *et al.* Energy requirement and physical activity in free-living older men and women: a doubly labeled water study. *J Appl Physiol* 1998; 85: 1036–1069.

3

The cost and the diseases

Obesity is an independent risk factor for major diseases, including coronary heart disease, type 2 diabetes mellitus and cancers (mainly breast cancer and cancer of the colon, kidney and oesophagus). It also contributes to the increased prevalence of other conditions, such as osteoarthritis, gallstones, infertility and gynaecological problems. In addition to the direct medical impact it also has a significant social impact, particularly in leading to low self-esteem, depression and social exclusion. Obesity can also result in respiratory disorders, particularly obstructive sleep apnoea syndrome, liver disease and skin conditions, some of which are rare and unique to obese individuals.[1]

The US Centers for Disease Control and Prevention (CDC) estimate that approximately 280 000 Americans die every year as a direct result of their excess weight. The annual healthcare cost in the US resulting from obesity is now approaching $240 billion, ironically at a time when Americans are spending $33 billion on various weight-loss schemes.[2] In the UK the National Audit Office suggests that there are 30 000 deaths per year caused by obesity and that life expectancy, in people who die as a result of their obesity, is shortened by an average of 9 years.[3]

In terms of disease risk and cost to the health system, obesity is a hugely important public health problem. Individuals who are overweight and remain overweight are more likely to have a range of conditions that will impact on their health and well-being, put them at increased risk of developing disease and ultimately increase their risk of early death. Health services will also suffer as resources become stretched to support overweight and obese patients and indeed this was the conclusion of the 2007 Foresight Report[4] which projected forward to 2050 when it estimated that if nothing is done, most adults will be obese and healthcare costs will bankrupt our society. Derek Wanless, in his reports to the UK government[5] on how the National Health Service will be funded in the future, came to a similar conclusion when he identified the considerable burden from disease resulting directly from a high prevalence of obesity.

Being overweight or obese significantly increases the risk of developing and dying from a range of conditions and these are summarised in box 3.1 and figure 3.1.

> *Box 3.1* Medical risks associated with overweight (BMI >25)
> populations[6]
>
> - high blood pressure, hypertension
> - abnormal blood cholesterol, dyslipidaemia
> - type 2 diabetes
> - insulin resistance, glucose intolerance
> - hyperinsulinaemia
> - coronary heart disease
> - congestive heart failure
> - stroke
> - gallstones
> - cholecystitis and cholelithiasis
> - gout
> - osteoarthritis
> - obstructive sleep apnoea and respiratory problems
> - some types of cancer (such as endometrial, breast, prostate, and colon)
> - complications of pregnancy
> - poor female reproductive health (such as polycystic ovary syndrome, menstrual irregularities, infertility, irregular ovulation)
> - bladder control problems (such as stress incontinence)
> - uric acid nephrolithiasis
> - psychological disorders (such as depression, eating disorders, distorted body image and low self-esteem).

For obese individuals the relative risk of disease is different for different conditions and these are summarised in table 3.1,[7] and the benefits of losing weight are summarised in table 3.2.[8]

Type 2 diabetes mellitus

Obesity is a major risk factor for development of type 2 diabetes. Considering that the proportion of people of European origin with a genetic predisposition to developing type 2 diabetes is between 30% and 50% it becomes clear that in an environment conducive to the development of diabetes – easy access to high-energy foods and little need for exercise – then the prevalence will increase rapidly. It has been established that lifestyle will hugely influence the number of individuals who go on to develop the disease and this can be seen in a number of population-based studies. The Pima Indians, a population with a high genetic predisposition to diabetes, and

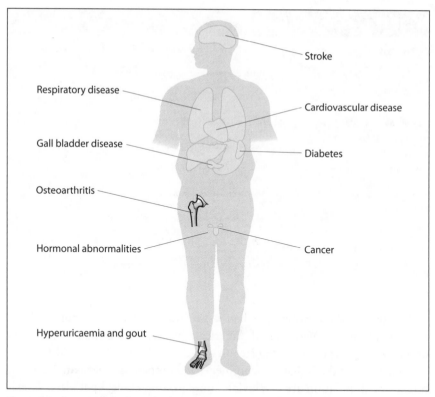

Figure 3.1 Impact of obesity on body systems.

who originate in a region that includes modern day Mexico, have an indigenous prevalence of diabetes that is relatively low. In their natural environment, their lifestyle is characterised by high levels of physical activity

Table 3.1 Relative risk of disease in obesity		
	Risk in women	**Risk in men**
Type 2 diabetes	12.7	5.2
Hypertension	4.2	2.6
Myocardial infarct	3.2	1.5
Colon cancer	2.7	3.0
Angina	1.8	1.8
Gall bladder disease	1.8	1.8
Ovarian cancer	1.7	–
Osteoarthritis	1.4	1.9
Stroke	1.3	1.3

Table 3.2 Benefits of 10% weight loss	
Mortality	>20% Decrease in total mortality
	>30% Decrease in diabetes-related deaths
	>40% Decrease in obesity-related deaths
Blood pressure	Decrease of 10 mmHg systolic
	Decrease of 20 mmHg diastolic
Diabetes	50% Decrease in fasting glucose
Lipids	10% Decrease total cholesterol
	15% Decrease in low-density lipoprotein
	30% Decrease in triglycerides
	8% Increase in high-density lipoprotein

From Jung.[8]

and a low-fat diet. However when a genetically identical group of Pima Indians adopted a Westernised American lifestyle in South Dakota, they developed a prevalence of diabetes that is the highest in the world.[9]

Likewise, on the Indian subcontinent, where there has been an economic boom, the population are displaying an interesting clinical paradox. This is an area mostly associated with famine, poverty and malnutrition and among the poor the incidence of type 2 diabetes has been traditionally low. Yet there is an increasing prevalence of diabetes in the middle classes, as this social group take on the trappings of middle-class wealth. Type 2 diabetes is the ultimate expression of the gene-environment interaction: 'Genetics loads the gun; the environment pulls the trigger'.[9]

What is perhaps more interesting is that since low birthweight is a predicator of central intra-abdominal fat accumulation in later life and a key component of the metabolic syndrome, of which diabetes is the ultimate result, low birthweight may be a factor that is exacerbating the obesity epidemic in India. With the existing genetic predisposition in the Indian population and the poverty of a generation ago when birthweights were often low, this offers a possible explanation, but sadly not a solution, to the sudden explosion in the prevalence of the disease in that part of the world.

Body fat is the main modifiable factor in the development of type 2 diabetes but other factors include:

- a pro-diabetic genetic endowment
- fetal undernutrition or stress resulting in low birthweight
- low infant growth
- low adult height

- physical inactivity
- high total fat content
- high intra-abdominal fat accumulation.

With a high genetic susceptibility to diabetes, the key to maximising the expression of the disease within a population boils down to two key factors: physical inactivity and obesity. Both are linked to lifestyle and simply push the energy balance into the black.

There is a growing body of evidence that simple lifestyle interventions can cut the incidence of type 2 diabetes.[10] By simply reducing daily energy intake and increasing exercise moderately, the incidence of type 2 diabetes fell by as much as 50%. This is significant and justifies a considerable investment in preventative strategies within the population.

Cancer

The Million Women Study followed one million women aged 50–64 years for seven years. In this time 45 000 were diagnosed with cancer and 17 000 of them died from the disease.[11] The study found that being overweight doubled the risk of certain cancers in women. In Britain's largest study of the link between weight and malignant disease, it was found that increasing obesity in the UK and the Western world is resulting in the increasing prevalence in cancer cases. Of 17 forms of cancer studied, an increase in BMI increased the risk of 10 forms. Being overweight accounts for 1 in 20 cancers or 6000 of the 120 000 cases diagnosed each year.

Half of the 6000 cases of endometrial cancer found each year are caused by the patient being overweight or obese. Excess weight is a risk factor in one type of oesophageal cancer. It is also found to increase the risk of kidney cancer, leukaemia, multiple myeloma, pancreatic cancer, non-Hodgkin's lymphoma, ovarian cancer, primary liver cancer and, in some age groups, breast and bowel cancer.[12]

Two-thirds of the additional 6000 cancers each year that are caused by overweight or obesity are uterine or breast cancers. The mechanisms by which obesity causes breast cancer is related to oestrogen, and abnormalities in the hormonal axis caused by peripheral conversion in adipose tissue. The exact relationship between obesity and breast cancer risk is complex; in postmenopausal women, and in the elderly, there is a positive correlation between the two conditions, whereas before the menopause, excess body weight has an inverse relationship with breast cancer risk. Because of the difficulty of effective breast examination in the obese state, excess weight is also related to the presence of more advanced disease at diagnosis and therefore a poor prognosis in both premenopausal and postmenopausal breast cancer. These results are summarised in table 3.3.[12]

Table 3.3 Increased risk of cancer from obesity in postmenopausal women not taking hormone replacement therapy

Cancer	Increased risk (%)*
Uterus	189
Oesophagus	138
Bowel (premenopausal)	61
Kidney	53
Leukaemia	50
Breast	40
Bone	31
Pancreas	24
Non-Hodgkin's lymphoma	17
Ovarian	14

*Calculated as percentage increase in risk in women with a BMI of 35 kg/m^2 compared with women with a BMI of 25 kg/m^2.

The World Cancer Research Fund Study[12] used analysis of 7000 cancer studies, which showed that processed meats such as salami, ham and bacon were such a risk factor for bowel cancer that they should be cut out completely. The key recommendation was that intake of red meat should be reduced to 500 g a week.

The risk of endometrial cancer is increased by the presence of overweight or obesity. Yo-yo dieting, in particular, and weight cycling magnify the effect, as do inactivity and a high-energy diet, independent of BMI.

It should also be remembered that cancer survival rates in women are reduced by the presence of obesity, which also increases the complications from surgery and radiotherapy. In men, it is unclear whether or not obesity increases the outright risk of prostate cancer, but it seems to have an adverse impact upon its detection and outcome. Obese men presenting with prostate cancer tend to have more severe pathological features and have higher relapse rates.

In addition, in the male, increased body weight and BMI have an increased risk of colon cancer which is not seen in women, possibly because of differences in fat distribution or to the use of hormone replacement therapy (HRT) in women, which has the benefit of lowering the risk. An increased waist circumference, however, is associated with raised colon cancer risk in both sexes.

Primary renal cell cancer accounts for 2% of all new cancer cases worldwide, and is rising steadily. Smoking and obesity are the main causal risk factors, accounting for approximately 20–30% of renal cell cancers. Hypertension, possibly as a result of obesity, may influence renal cell cancer development, by an unknown mechanism.

Alcohol, tobacco and obesity act synergistically in increasing levels of hepatocellular carcinoma and adenocarcinoma of the lower oesophagus and gastric cardia.

Obesity is also implicated in the risk of pancreatic cancer, possibly because of increased refined carbohydrate intake, insulin resistance, hyperinsulinaemia and physical inactivity.

Cardiovascular disease

Cardiovascular disease (CVD) is prevalent throughout the UK and globally. Within the UK the good news is that there has been a 30% decrease in the incidence of cardiovascular disease deaths over the past 10 years but the prevalence still remains high with more than one in three people dying from CVD (39%) – the overall number of deaths are just over 238 000 per year.[13] However, the increasing incidence of type 2 diabetes, a major independent risk factor for coronary heart disease (CHD) and stroke, and closely linked to obesity, is likely to herald a rise in its prevalence. As CHD and stroke mortality in association with obesity take time to develop, it is not yet reflected in the current mortality figures. As the obesity epidemic has been a product of the past 30 years, the average obese person is yet to reach the age of premature death, however, over the next two decades as the obese population ages, rates are set to rise dramatically. Even if prevention of obesity is 100% successful, and not one person in the UK gains any more weight, there are sufficient obese individuals currently to make deaths from CHD inevitable.

The Interheart[14] study looked at 15 000 individuals worldwide who had their first myocardial infarction (MI), and compared them with 15 000 matched controls, in order to discover which of nine modifiable risk factors were most closely associated with CHD risk. As expected, cholesterol was confirmed as the major factor, with smoking another serious driver but abdominal obesity was identified as the major factor for MI in 20% of cases and being partly to blame in 34%.

A moderate increase of 5–10% in body weight in adulthood is associated with a 1.5 times increase in relative risk of death from coronary heart disease and non-fatal myocardial infarction and this increase in risk applies where the weight is maintained at the higher end of the normal range. The facts are alarming even in females where the risk of CHD is lower: an increase of 9 kg from teenage years to middle-age doubles the woman's risk of suffering a heart attack.[15]

Increased body fat is an independent risk factor for risk of heart disease and is equivalent to that associated with cigarette smoking, hypertension and elevated blood lipids. Increased body fat increases the risk of low-grade inflammation of the inner lining of arterial vessels and this inflammation increases the risk of MI and stroke. In addition obesity has been identified as an independent risk for congestive heart failure.[15]

Weight gain after age 18 years markedly increases the risk of hypertension compared with those who do not increase weight, and similarly, increases in total serum cholesterol and triglycerides result from increased body fat. Conversely, a 5–10% weight loss often normalises an obese person's serum cholesterol and triglycerides and reduces blood pressure as well as overall risk of heart disease, including risk of congestive heart failure. Indeed, the tendency to increase weight with age seems to explain the relationship between age and blood pressure. The 7-year study of Harvard alumni showed that men with a body weight 20% or more above 'desirable weight' experience a death rate 2.5 times higher than the leanest men. There is little question that obesity has been identified as an independent risk factor for coronary heart disease and is of a similar scale to cigarette smoking, hypertension, raised cholesterol and sedentary lifestyle.[15]

Metabolic syndrome

Metabolic syndrome describes a cluster of cardiometabolic risk factors associated with abdominal obesity. It is a clinical state that defines an individual's particular risk of developing both type 2 diabetes and cardiovascular disease. The International Diabetes Federation[16] has defined metabolic syndrome as:

- central obesity: waist circumference >94 cm in males or >80 cm in females
- raised total triglycerides: >1.7 mmol/L
- reduced high-density lipoproteins (HDLs): <1.03 mmol/L for males; <1.29 mmol/L for females
- blood pressure: >130 mmHg systolic and >85 mmHg diastolic
- raised fasting blood glucose: >5.6 mmol/L.

The strict definitions of the metabolic syndrome have attracted a great deal of controversy. On the one hand, they are criticised for overlooking other crucial factors that arise as a result of the same metabolic profile: conditions such as hypercoagulability of the blood, non-alcoholic steatohepatitis and polycystic ovarian syndrome. These issues would certainly add further complexity to the metabolic syndrome and could, because of this complexity, reduce its usefulness and its management. On the other hand, some physicians perhaps cynically accept this point and suggest that metabolic syndrome is really only a polite or more clinical way of telling a patient that they are too fat.[17]

There is good evidence that interventions to improve these clinical parameters can reduce the risk of developing CHD and type 2 diabetes. Obesity, more specifically central obesity, is therefore an independent risk factor for cardiovascular and metabolic disease – a cardiometabolic risk factor.

Fertility

Maternity deaths in Britain increased over the three years from 2004 to 2007 and one of the key factors suspected in contributing to this rise is obesity.[18] Others include older mothers giving birth, and the drive towards home or natural births. More mothers died during pregnancy and childbirth in 2003–2005 than in 2000–2002.[19]

The Confidential Enquiry into Maternal and Child Health (CEMACH) has reported that obesity is a key factor in the risk of death among new mothers.[19] Almost 300 women died after childbirth between 2003 and 2005 – with over half of the victims overweight. The CEMACH report claims that 40% of the deaths were avoidable.

The British Fertility Society have warned that fertility care may be rationed for obese women and that they should be refused treatment for infertility until they lose weight.[18] This restriction on treatment is necessary for women's safety and to ensure that the treatment had the maximum chance of success. The society suggested that treatment should be banned in women with a BMI of more than 35 kg/m².

A study has shown that maternal obesity is associated with doubling of the risk of stillbirth,[20] yet this study did not provide information regarding absolute risk. Neither did it evaluate to what extent this association may be explained by other known risk factors for adverse perinatal outcomes that are frequently seen in obese women, such as hypertension and diabetes.

Polycystic ovary syndrome is defined by the Rotterdam consensus as comprising two out of three of:

- clinical or biochemical signs of hyperandrogenism – acne, hirsutism, alopecia or a raised testosterone on blood testing
- oligo- or amenorrhoea – absent or reduced number of periods
- polycystic ovaries on ultrasound

There is a strong link with insulin resistance, even in lean individuals with the syndrome, and a close relationship with type 2 diabetes. It is associated with dietary obstacles, such as sweet cravings, bulimia nervosa, central adiposity, and low cholecystokinin (the satiety peptide).[21]

Obesity and mental health

The link between obesity and depression has long been assumed but there has never been any significant depth of evidence to define this link absolutely. What is not easily established is whether obesity or depression came first in the cycle of weight gain and low self-esteem. Equally controversial is the psychological effect of dieting: beneficial, by alleviating the stresses associated with obesity, or harmful, by accentuating anxieties and self-loathing when the almost inevitable recidivism occurs. There is no conclusive current evidence to support the hypothesis that obese people exhibit a higher level of mental illness than people of normal weight.[22] However, a major American study demonstrated that obesity in women increases the risk of major depression by 37% but obesity in men was shown to reduce the equivalent risk by 37%, whereas in men it was underweight that was linked with markedly higher risks of depression and suicide, possibly because depressed men smoked more heavily. A recent National Obesity Forum poll revealed that over half of overweight people – in particular young women – lack self-confidence because of their weight, most notably when swimming, exercising, on holiday or in public houses. Forty-one per cent felt that they were judged more because of their weight than anything else; 25% had experienced insults from children. Conversely a third of the 'lean' population admitted to treating overweight people differently from others, and a quarter believe that overweight people simply lacked control. The same poll revealed that the majority of overweight people realise not only the fact of their overweight, but that weight is not merely a cosmetic issue, but a health matter. Sixty per cent of overweight people admitted that their health was affected by being overweight; 63% thought lack of exercise was the problem, and 55% thought that a poor diet was a contributory factor.[23]

A subset of overweight patients has been identified who display frequent episodes of binge eating and increased levels of psychological stress. Another eating disorder, night eating syndrome, is a well-known pattern of disturbed eating and is also related to obesity, and induces elevated scores on measures of depressive illness. Patients suffering from binge eating disorder display features of bulimia nervosa, without the compensatory features inducing weight loss such as purging, vomiting or abnormal exercise regimes. Its features include:

- recurrent episodes of eating objectively large amounts of food within a discrete period of time and by a subjective sense of lack of control during each episode. The episodes are associated with three or more of the following:

- eating much more rapidly than normal
- eating until feeling uncomfortably full
- eating large amounts of food when not feeling physically hungry
- eating alone because of being embarrassed by how much one is eating
- feeling disgusted with oneself, depressed, or very guilty after overeating
- marked distress about the binge eating behaviour
- binge eating, on average, at least 2 days per week for 6 months
- binge eating not associated with the regular use of inappropriate compensatory behaviours (e.g., purging, fasting, excessive exercise).

Some studies show that 2.5% of adult women, and 1.1% of men have binge eating disorder, of whom most but not all are obese, and it is crucial that these individuals are picked up at the earliest possible stage of the treatment pathway, as traditional remedies will be unsuccessful unless the fundamental underlying psychopathology is addressed. The treatment of the disorder is usually weight management but with the addition of cognitive behavioural therapy. Strict diet regimes including meal replacements and low- or very-low-energy diets, as well as over-the-counter remedies should be avoided as they are likely to aggravate the condition. Cognitive behavioural therapy helps patients to develop normal behaviour patterns aimed at regaining the control of eating; weight management is unlikely to succeed without it.

Night eating syndrome, like binge eating, is also associated with psychological and emotional factors. Patients may be moody, tense, anxious, nervous and depressed, and as with binge eating disorder, they must be identified accurately and quickly, as standard remedies will not only fail in the long term, but also be harmful to individuals.

Symptoms and criteria include:

- morning anorexia, i.e. no appetite for breakfast; the first food of the day is delayed by several hours
- evening hyperphagia, i.e. excess food in the evening; 50% of the day's intake is eaten after the end of the evening meal and after 7 p.m.
- a pattern that has persisted for at least 2 months
- guilt feelings while eating; eating causes tension and anxiety, not enjoyment
- frequent waking during the night, usually with eating during waking intervals
- eating mainly carbohydrates and sugars at inappropriate times
- continuous eating during the evening, unlike binge eating disorder, in which eating is in short episodes.

Prevalence in the population is around 1–2%, rising to 10% of obese patients, and as many as a quarter of grossly obese people. It is associated with obstructive sleep apnoea and restless leg syndrome. Most patients are said to have eaten fast and carelessly, with 30% having injured themselves owing to overzealous eating behaviour. The most appropriate and potentially successful management is based around behavioural rather than dietary therapy, inducing patients to have an early, substantial breakfast, and regain a normal eating pattern.[24]

In society, obesity is associated with considerable stigma, with obese people subjected to public disproval on a daily basis. There is good evidence that employers will discriminate against obese people in job interviews, and that obese individuals achieve less in terms of education, work, social interactions and relationships.

Respiratory conditions

It is generally accepted that conditions such as asthma, emphysema, and chronic obstructive pulmonary disease are made worse by obesity, simply because of the extra mechanical and metabolic effort required to perform the tasks of daily living. There is, however, a vicious circle in place, as these respiratory conditions also limit the amount of exercise such individuals can attain, inducing more sedentary lifestyles, further driving obesity levels upwards.

Sleep apnoea

Excess fat deposited in the neck, chest wall and abdomen has adverse effects on lung function. Apnoeic episodes can lead to pulmonary hypertension, myocardial stress, excessive daytime drowsiness and altered tissue oxygenation during the night.[24]

Obesity has long been known to cause sleep apnoea. People who suffer from obstructive sleep apnoea breathe shallowly or stop breathing for short periods while sleeping. This can happen many times during the night. It results in poor sleep, leading to excessive sleepiness during the day. Because these events occur during sleep, a person with sleep apnoea is often the last one to know what is happening. The initial assessment of sleep apnoea is by a simple questionnaire called the Epworth sleep score, which describes eight common scenarios (such as sitting as a passenger in a car for over an hour) each of which attracts a score between 0 and 3 corresponding to the likelihood of falling asleep in that situation. The higher the score, the greater the daytime somnolence, and subsequently the chances of a diagnosis of sleep apnoea, necessitating formal sleep studies. It is worth considering that this daytime somnolence, which is strongly associated with accidental deaths and road traffic accidents, is most common in sedentary professions such as drivers of heavy-goods vehicles, taxis and buses, so its identification is essential.

In deep sleep, the muscles of the throat relax. Normally this does not cause any problems with breathing. In sleep apnoea, complete relaxation of the throat muscles causes blockage of the upper airway at the back of the tongue. Normal breathing then slows or stops completely. Such an episode is called an apnoeic episode. During an episode, people with obstructive sleep apnoea make constant efforts to breath against their blocked airway until the blood oxygen level begins to fall. The brain then needs to arouse the person from deep, relaxed sleep so that the muscle tone returns, the upper airway then opens and breathing begins again. This can be repeated a number of times during the night.

The simplest treatment to manage sleep apnoea is to lose weight. If this is unsuccessful or these measures are not enough, the best form of treatment is continuous positive airway pressure (CPAP) therapy in which a gentle flow of air is applied through the nose at night keeping the pressure in the throat above atmospheric pressure and stopping the throat narrowing to prevent breathing pauses and snoring.[25]

Skin diseases associated with obesity

Obesity has a significant impact on the skin resulting in dermatological conditions such as achrocordons, candidosis, cellulite and intertrigo.[26] They may result from an increased amount of skin or where the weight placed on the skin can contribute to the development of decubitus ulcers and plantar hyperkeratosis. Acanthosis nigricans is associated with certain malignancies and might indicate underlying physiological changes created by the obese state.

Among the most commonly encountered dermatoses in obese patients is acanthosis nigricans (AN) a blacking of the skin in certain regions of the body; however, it cannot be predicted which obese patient will be affected. While classically associated with an underlying malignancy, AN appears to be tightly linked to diabetes and obesity. This is explained by the observations that obese patients have higher levels of insulin than people who are not obese. The foundations of AN are cellular insulin resistance, increased insulin production, stimulation of insulin-like growth factor (IGF) receptors by insulin and IGF-receptor induction of keratinocyte proliferation. This results in a thickening of the skin and no change in pigmentation. The relative velvety darkness on the nape and under the breasts is due to hyperkeratosis. AN was observed in 74% of patients with obesity, with patients who are of African-American descent having a higher incidence than white patients.[26]

Yeast infections, as would be expected, are a very common problem among the obese. The maceration and moisture found in skinfold areas provide an ideal environment for the proliferation of yeasts, such as *Candida* leading to redness and irritation, with the characteristic satellite lesions under the breasts, under the abdominal fold and in the inguinal area.

The cobblestone appearance of the buttocks and thighs occurs more frequently in obese women than in obese men, almost by definition because of the increased body mass and skin. The cause is unclear but involves the microcirculation and lymphatics with the fat pushing through the framework of the superficial fascia.

Decubitus ulcers appear to be more prevalent in obese patients who spend above average time on their backs. Whether this is due to increased pressure on the capillaries or kinking of the blood supply caused by the excessive weight impinging upon the vessels is not clear. Wound healing also appears to be slower in the obese patient. Owing to the increased girth there are great problems in the healing of surgical wounds.

Psoriasis occurs more frequently in obese patients, but the reasons for this are unclear. The evidence is indirect, in that weight-reduction programmes can diminish the severity of psoriasis in the obese patient. Both the psoriatic patient and the obese patient have common co-morbidities, including cardiovascular disease, depression, type 2 diabetes mellitus, dyslipidaemia, and hypertension; however, there are no studies that can confirm the association between the two.

Chronic stasis dermatitis can also lead to elephantiasis. Excessive amounts of bodyweight place an obvious strain upon the legs. Treatment with support stockings further emphasises the role of obesity in the development of stasis dermatitis and stasis ulceration.

Musculoskeletal conditions

It is unsurprising that musculoskeletal conditions such as osteoarthritis of the hips and knees are increased, purely by dint of the extra mechanical burden induced by excess weight. Prosthetic knee and hip joints perform less well, and indeed are not guaranteed in the presence of obesity because of the likelihood of mechanical failure. Gout is significantly more common in the presence of obesity. However, it is less intuitive to learn that the condition of non-weight-bearing joints such as the wrists is also adversely affected, suggesting a metabolic cause for joint inflammation related to the obesity.

Possibly the most important musculoskeletal condition related to obesity, in terms of its effect on the economy and productivity in the workforce is low-back pain; excess weight leading to extra load on the back is implicated in its cause. The root cause in many cases is spinal shrinkage, a result of compressive forces resulting in compression of vertebral discs. Pressure on the discs is reduced in the lying position leading to an increase in spinal length, and the reduction in the length of the spine on standing, leading to low-back pain, under the influence of obesity is defined as spinal shrinkage. Forty per cent of body length is taken up by the spine, of which one-third is represented by intervertebral discs the height of which varies, depending on the forces applied. Reduction in levels of obesity diminishes the abnormal stresses on the spine, reducing back pain, and increasing functionality.[27]

Liver disease

Liver disease, especially in the form of non-alcoholic steatohepatitis (NASH) is becoming increasingly common as a consequence of the rising prevalence of obesity. NASH is set to become one of the most common causes of end-stage liver failure, because of its progression from benign non-alcoholic fatty liver disease to cirrhosis, portal hypertension and hepatocellular carcinoma. The liver changes observed in alcoholic liver disease are typical of NASH but the developmental factors are obesity, diabetes, hyperlipidaemia and hypertension. Obesity and insulin resistance are major factors in NASH, which is generally asymptomatic, although some individuals may describe tiredness and abdominal discomfort; hepatomegaly occurs in up to 75% of patients, but other signs of liver disease are rare. The prevalence of NASH is between 2% and 9% of the population, of whom 50% will develop fibrosis, 30% will develop cirrhosis, and 3% end up with liver failure or transplantation.

There is also a strong connection between gallbladder disease and obesity.

Mortality

It seems that the theory that fat is bad and more fat is worse is perhaps not as clear-cut as was first thought and some recent research is now challenging this orthodoxy. A study by the US Centers for Disease Control and Prevention[28] suggests that being overweight (BMI 25–30 kg/m^2) might not be associated with as negative a health consequence as was initially predicted. It showed that overweight people have a higher risk of dying from kidney disease and diabetes compared with people of normal weight but a lower risk of dying from a range of conditions including emphysema, pneumonia and lung disease. It also found that overweight people are no more likely to die from heart disease and cancer than those of normal weight.

Interesting this research suggests that people classified as overweight have a lower mortality rate than those who are underweight, obese or normal. The study confirms that obese people have higher death rates compared with

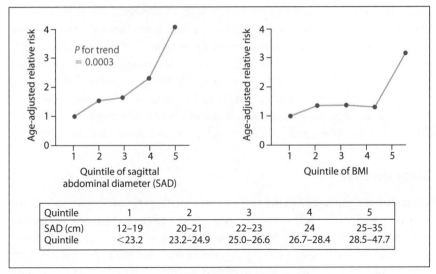

Quintile	1	2	3	4	5
SAD (cm)	12–19	20–21	22–23	24	25–35
Quintile	<23.2	23.2–24.9	25.0–26.6	26.7–28.4	28.5–47.7

Figure 3.2 Paris Prospective Study. Reproduced from Fontbonne and Eschwege[29] with permission.

non-obese people but that this is driven mainly by deaths caused by CHD; deaths from cancer are similar between these groups.

The Paris Prospective Study[29] showed that sudden death is dramatically increased in the presence of obesity (figure 3.2).

Certain cancers are associated with being obese: colon, breast, kidney and pancreas cancers resulted in higher death rates in obese patients compared with normal-weight patients but this was not shown for overweight people.

What this CDC study does suggest is that being overweight does not seem to increase mortality risk and therefore would not support a recommendation for those in this group to lose weight. Clearly this finding further complicates the details of national guidance on obesity. Yet the study must be taken in context as it focused on mortality, not on disease incidence, and it could be postulated that an individual who contracts a disease and who is overweight might be more likely to survive that disease; being overweight offers additional resources to deal with the disease. Yet even given this, some of the graphs in the World Cancer Research Fund Study[12] suggest that not only is there no difference in mortality rates from cancers between normal-weight and overweight individuals, there is also no difference in the incidence in cancers between these groups, adding support to the CDC study. Data from the CDC study suggests no increased risk of dying from heart disease in overweight individuals.

So what might this study mean? Good health is more than not dying and the CDC study is exclusively a study of dying. For this reason it is unlikely that the study will radically affect the health messages currently agreed on healthy weight targets. It remains clear that those who are overweight are more likely to have CHD, type 2 diabetes, gallstones, high blood pressure and some types of cancers. Indeed the processes that leads to cancer and results in death in obese individuals might begin when the individual is overweight only to show up much later in life. The message for the overweight may be to eat healthily and take exercise rather than focus on losing weight. Of course it is also vital that all individuals must guard against overweight slipping into obesity.

Conclusion

Obesity is a major cause of morbidity and premature mortality and, as a result, is a major drain on national healthcare resources. Whereas it causes and worsens a large number of conditions, the main concern is the impact of obesity in the development of type 2 diabetes and the impact that this will have on rates of coronary heart disease. Studies predict that the increase in diabetes and other chronic diseases driven by the prevalence of obesity, could lead to a fall in general life expectancy. Olshansky and colleagues[30] in 2005 warned that life expectancy could be cut by 5 years in the coming decades if obesity continues to increase and in this way we might witness a turnaround in the year-on-year increase experienced from the early 1900s up to the present day. This is indeed a sobering thought.

References

1. World Health Organization/Food & Agricultural Organization. *Diet, Nutrition and the Prevention of Chronic Diseases.* WHO Technical Report Series 916. Geneva: WHO/FAO, 2003.
2. Cannon G. *Dieting Makes You Fat.* Virgin Books, 2008.
3. National Audit Office. *Tackling Obesity in England.* London: The Stationary Office, 2001.
4. King M *et al. Foresight Project Report. Tackling Obesities: future choices.* London: Government Office For Science, 2007.
5. Wanless D. *Securing Good Health for the Whole Population.* London: HM Treasury, 2004.
6. Waddden T, Stunkard A. *Handbook of Obesity Treatment.* London: Guilford Press, 2002.
7. World Health Organization. *Obesity: preventing and managing the global epidemic.* WHO Technical Report Series 894 (3) I-253. Geneva: WHO, 2003.
8. Jung R. Obesity as a disease. *Br Med Bull* 1997; 53: 307–321.
9. Van Gaal L. *Managing Obesity and Diabetes.* London: Science Press, 2003.
10. Knowler, W C *et al.* Reduction in the incidence of type 2 diabetes with lifestyle intervention or metformin. *N Eng J Med* 2002; 346: 393–403.
11. Reeves G *et al.* Cancer incidence and mortality in relation to body mass index in the Million Women Study: cohort study. *BMJ* 2007; 335: 1134.
12. World Cancer Research Fund. *Food, Nutrition, Physical Activity, and Prevention of Cancer: a global perspective.* Washington: DCO AICR, 2007.
13. Department of Health. *Choosing Health: making healthier choices easier.* London: Department of Health, 2004.

14. Yusuf S *et al.* Effect of potentially modifiable risk factors associated with myocardial infarction in 52 countries (the INTERHEART Study): A case control study. *Lancet* 2004; 364: 937–952.
15. Bray G. Health hazard of obesity. *Endo Metabol Clin N Am* 1985; 25: 907–919.
16. Grundy S *et al.* Definition of metabolic syndrome. *Circulation* 2004; 109: 433–438.
17. Byrne C, Wade S, eds. *The Metabolic Syndrome.* Chichester: John Wiley, 2005.
18. Confidential Enquiry into Maternal and Child Health. *Obesity in Pregnancy Audit.* http://www.cemach.org.uk (accessed Feb 2009). London: CEMACH, 2008.
19. Chu SY, Kim SY *et al.* Maternal obesity and risk of stillbirth: a metaanalysis. *Am J Obstet Gynecol* 2007; 197: 223–228.
20. Confidential Inquiry Into Maternal and Child Health. *Risk of Stillbirth and Obesity.* London: CEMACH, 2004.
21. Hirschberg AL *et al.* Impaired cholecystokinin secretion and disturbed appetite regulation in women with polycystic ovary syndrome. *Gynecol Endocrinol* 2004; 19: 79–87.
22. O'Shea A. Obesity and its management. *Irish Pharm*; Mar 2008.
23. Haslam D. *Obesity: your questions answered.* Oxford: Radcliffe Medical Press, 2006.
24. Samuaels M. Medical and psychiatric co-morbidities in obese women with and without binge eating disorder. *Int J Eat Disord* 2002; 32: 72–78.
25. Trenell MI *et al.* Influence of constant positive airway pressure therapy on lipid storage, muscle metabolism and insulin action in obese patients with severe obstructive sleep apnoea syndrome. *Diabetes Obes Metab* 2007; 9: 679–687.
26. Scheinfeld N S *et al. Expert Rev Dermatol* 2007; 2: 409–415.
27. Van Dieen J H, Toussaint H M. Spinal shrinkage as a parameter of functional load. *Spine* 1993; 18: 1504–1514.
28. Flegal K *et al.* Cause-specific excess death associated with underweight, overweight, and obesity. *JAMA* 2007; 298: 2028–2037.
29. Fontbonne AM, Eschwege EM. Insulin and cardiovascular disease: Paris Prospective Study. *Diabetes Care* 1991; 14: 461–469.
30. Olshansky S *et al.* A potential decline in life expectancy in the United States of America in the 21st Century. *N Engl J Med* 2005; 352: 1138–1142.

4

Public health and the politics of food

With regard to our health, we have a lot to be proud of. At the beginning of the 20th century, average life expectancy in Britain was under 50 years. Infant mortality was approximately 150 per 1000 births. Among the poorer sectors of the population, over 200 infants in every 1000 born alive in 1900 died in their first year of life. Today, by contrast, average life expectancy in Britain for men is 78 years and for women is 82 years and is set to rise. Of the 10 years of average life expectancy gained since the creation of the NHS in the late 1940s, about half has been derived from factors such as better food standards and collective protection from hazards such as infections and accidents. The other five additional life years have stemmed from better medicines and enhanced surgical techniques employed in individual care,[1] so we are doing pretty well.

In the past 100 years the distribution of diseases between different countries has historically reflected their degree of industrialisation. With increasing industrialisation, life expectancy increases, accompanied by a shift from infectious disease to degenerative disease as the most frequent cause of death. The determinants of health are many and wide-ranging and often interact with each other in complex ways.[2]

It has been estimated that successful smoking cessation, combined with dietary improvements such as an additional daily serving of fruit and vegetables, and a shift from inactivity to moderate activity, could potentially increase life expectancy by 11 years. That would be equivalent to closing the entire longevity gap between Britain's most and least advantaged groups, the core of social inequalities in health.[2]

Cardiovascular death rates, for example, climbed continuously between the 1870s and the 1950s, partly because the population had improving access to tobacco and fatty foods. Such goods are typically consumed in increasing quantities in communities that are in the process of becoming wealthy. Populations remaining very poor cannot afford them, while those who are rich and well educated tend to turn to less hazardous choices. We are witnessing this pattern occurring in a condensed time frame in countries such as Malta and Kuwait where, rather than taking 100 years to occur, staggeringly high levels of obesity are occurring over a 10–15 year period. In Mauritius from 1987 to 1992 the prevalence of people overweight increased by 10%. In Kuwait the prevalence of obesity at the beginning of the 1990s was as high as 32% in men and 41% in women.

It is not a time for complacency. As stated in Chapter 3, studies predict that the increase in diabetes, and other chronic diseases that are driven by the prevalence of obesity, could lead to a fall in general life expectancy by as much as 5 years in the coming decades if obesity continues to increase. Indeed we might witness a turnaround in the year-on-year increase in life expectancy that we achieved from the early 1900s up to the present day.[3]

Public health

Determinants of health

The Whitehead and Dahlgren model of the determinants of health (figure 4.1) shows that a person's health is determined by myriad factors.[5] At the centre of the model is the individual – dependent on genetic make up, sex and age, there will be a risk of developing specific diseases. For example, a man might be more likely to have type 2 diabetes mellitus compared with other males in his community because of his genetic make up.

His susceptibility to diabetes is also dependent on his lifestyle. If he is overweight because he consumes too many calories and takes little exercise then he is more likely to develop the disease.

Social and community networks are normally viewed in a positive way in that they influence more healthy lifestyles in the individual. They provide 'social capital' to support healthier choices and patient empowerment. However, 'cultural norms' can also have a negative impact on health. The diet in some Asian communities is very healthy as it is based on vegetarian foods whereas others are not, particularly where *ghee* (a type of butter fat used in cooking) is common, and where sugary confection, which in the past was seen as a treat for special occasions, is now often eaten on a daily basis. The 'Ulster fry' popular in Northern Ireland consists of a large amount of saturated fat; it is unhealthy but as it is a cultural norm it is difficult to convince individuals to change to more healthy foods. Perhaps a more bizarre cultural expression of unhealthy food is the deep fried Mars bar popular in some areas of Glasgow.

Further out from the individual in the Whitehead and Dahlgren model, (figure 4.1) education and agriculture policies have a direct impact on population health. In Finland in the 1970s, agriculture policy was changed to introduce low-fat options into the national diet.[6] Finnish people were traditionally dependent on foods high in saturated fats. This policy changed

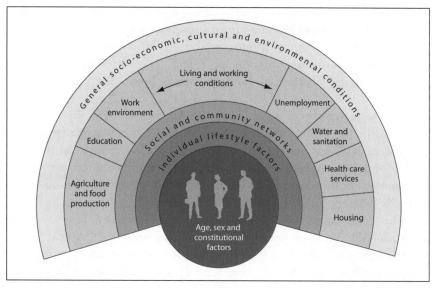

Figure 4.1 Determinants of health. Reproduced with permission from Dahlgren G, Whitehead M (1991). *Policies and Strategies to Promote Social Equity in Health*. Stockholm, Sweden: Institute for Futures Studies.

thanks to an intense public information campaign, resulting in a 20% reduction in the coronary heart disease (CHD) death rate in 10 years, so that Finland experienced an average, rather than its formerly high, CHD mortality rate. Their government's policy included: paying dividends to dairy farmers for producing low-fat options; creating wider choices for the consumer; and promoting an understanding of the issues through public information campaigns, allowing people to be able to choose a healthier diet.

The more educated a community is, the more likely its members are to be in employment and the more likely they will be to make healthy choices for themselves and their dependents.

The Whitehead and Dahlgren model articulates the complexity of human health and outlines the range of actions required to support good health within communities. Some of this will be down to the individuals, the family and the community, whereas some will be due to local and national government regulation.

Nutrition

In May 2008 a national newspaper in the UK reported on a public survey under the title 'Confusion over official advice on healthy diet'.[7] The survey of 1347 people suggested considerable confusion among the public on what was meant by 'five portions a day' in the government programme on healthy eating of fruit and vegetables. This is hardly surprising given the conflicting and confusing messages emerging from a food industry with a central objective to get people to consume more and more of its products. The Sugar Bureau, the publicity organisation for Tate & Lyle and British Sugar, still publish promotional material for UK doctors promoting the benefits of sugar.[8]

The prosperity of post-war Europe and America brought unprecedented freedoms. In 1954 food rationing ended in the UK, spawning a generation of children with few restrictions with regard to food intake, in terms of quality or quantity. Food was produced and eaten with little concern about its impact on health. Most information about nutrition came from slimming manuals that appeared in the 1960s – often strongly opposed to carbohydrates, condemning them as foods that should be avoided. Professor John Yudkin's book *This Slimming Business*, first published in 1958, was hostile to carbohydrate foods suggesting that they should be avoided, particularly by individuals wishing to lose weight. Professor Yudkin saw both starches and sugar as similar in effect.

Short history of food policy

The first real attempt to define a healthy national diet was the McGovern report, *Dietary Goals for the United States* published in 1977,[9] which proved hugely influential in changing the dietary habits of Americans. Senator George McGovern's report made a sharp distinction between sugar and starches and their respective impacts on health. The report identified that processed foods containing fats, sugar and salt were being widely and aggressively promoted to the public, whereas food rich in wholegrain, fruit and vegetable were seldom advertised. This had resulted in a massive decline in the consumption of these foods over a 30-year period since the end of the Second World War. The McGovern report also highlighted the concern that processed foods often contained few vitamins and minerals, and thus had little nutritional value beyond their, often considerable, calorific value. The McGovern report set out dietary goals that would form the basis of a national healthy eating policy. The McGovern recommendations are compared with the consumption of food elements in table 4.1.

At the time the McGovern report was being published in the US, a similar programme was being advanced in the UK. Persistence by a group of medical practitioners in the UK ensured publication of the 1983 Royal College of Physicians report on obesity, which described the huge public health implications of an emerging obesity epidemic.[10] Like the McGovern report, the RCP report made a clear distinction between starch and sugar, stressing the benefits of starchy foods as part of a healthy diet and emphasising that starch-based foods were not a key reason for obesity. They agreed with the

Table 4.1 Actual versus recommended consumption of food types in US, 1977		
	Total energy intake (%)	
	Actual	McGovern goal
Protein	12	12
Fat	42	30
Starch	22	40–45
Sugar	24	15

McGovern report on a reduction in fat from 42% to 30% but recommended halving calories from sugar to 12% of the total.

In 1979, the UK government, conscious of the link between diet and a range of degenerative diseases, set up the National Advisory Committee on Nutrition Education (NACNE) to report on nutritional improvement. The Committee consisted of nutritionists, health educationalists and representatives of the food industry. The committee was charged with making food information and nutritional advice clearer for the general public. It produced its first report in 1983 giving, for the first time, precise targets for dietary intake; these are roughly the targets that we have today.

The chairman of NACNE, Professor J N Morris, asked Professor Philip James to report on what guidelines the public should follow in choosing which foods to eat. James, with the help of other experts, produced his report in 1981 with conclusions that were broadly in line with those in the McGovern report and for the same reasons.

With a strong lobby from the food industry (the British Nutrition Foundation and the Food and Drinks Industries Council) sitting on the NACNE main committee, there was objection to the recommendations of the James Report. Although this form of lobbying could have been expected, what was not so clear at the time was why there was objection from the Department of Health representatives. It transpired that they were further influenced by the Ministry of Agriculture, Fisheries and Food, a strong supporter of British farmers and the food industry; this was government policy pursued strongly by a government department – yet acting against public health. Indeed this was the very problem that was addressed in Finland, where public health collaborated with agriculture to produce an impressive impact on public health for the Finnish population.

Professor James revised his report three times between 1980 and 1983 yet it was still rejected. The James report was, however, published as a discussion document by the Health Education Council alongside a refusal by the Department of Health to recognise most of its recommendations.

Table 4.2 Short-term and long-term nutritional guidelines proposed by NACNE, 1983

Dietary component	Short-term target	Long-term target
Energy		Energy intake to maintain optimal body weight, with exercise
Total fat	34% of energy	30% of energy
Saturated fat	Decrease to 15% of energy	Decrease to 10% of total energy
Polyunsaturated	Increase to 5% of total energy	No specific target; reduce saturated fat and polyunsaturated will rise
Sucrose	Decrease to 34 kg per head per year	Decrease to 20 kg per head per year
Dietary fibre	Increase to 25 g per head per day	Increase to 30 g per head per day
Salt	Reduce by 1 g per day	Reduce to 3 g per day
Alcohol	No more than 5% of energy	Levels should not exceed 4% of energy
Protein		Maintained, with a greater proportion coming from vegetable and protein sources

NACNE = National Advisory Committee on Nutrition Education.

These were included in the Royal College of Physician's report on obesity in 1983.[10] These are summarised in table 4.2.

The RCP report was ignored for 10 years, despite a government public health White Paper published by William Waldegrave on the topic. Things only happened, and the merits of Professor James's report recognised, when the Chief Medical Officer, Donald Acheson, set out Geoffrey Rose's concept of shifting the population distribution in relation to chronic disease.[11] To do this the obesity rates needed to be halved.

Politically, in the 1980s, ignoring a robust scientific assessment on nutritional needs was not unreasonable. Other seminal reports such as the Black report[12] had clearly established the existence of social and health inequalities and were more or less ignored by the government of the day, as much of what they recommended opposed commercial and other vested interests.

This was certainly true for the food industry which, like the tobacco industry, was well organised and a skilful advocate for its cause. However, unlike tobacco, food is essential to life, it is part of human culture and changes in diet are more difficult to bring about as the messages need to be clear and unambiguous and this often served the interests of the food industry.

Scotland was more amenable to giving a priority to obesity, producing the first Scottish Intercollegiate Guidelines Network (SIGN) guidelines on obesity management that adopted a community and monitoring approach and re-introduced the concept of waist measurements.[13] It was not warmly accepted by general practitioners who saw it as too time consuming and perhaps reflecting a certain conflict between public health and the practice of medicine. It was also ignored by central government in Whitehall but after the 1997 Labour election victory and extensive consultations by the World Health Organization (WHO), the newly elected Labour government commissioned Professor James to produce a report on the prevention of childhood obesity. The need for this work was supported by the Foods Standards report at the same time. Professor James's new report was wide-ranging in its recommendations but was largely attacked by the government as it presented some novel and politically unpalatable ideas about the marketing of energy-dense foods to schools, school foods and soft drink/confectionary issues and understandably these recommendations were strongly opposed by the major food producers.

Beyond Finland, the UK and the US, other nations were also beginning to address the impact of food policy on health. A key report by WHO[14] provided national governments with an international perspective on the emerging problem and on setting out ways of tackling it.

Of course it was now accepted that food standards needed to be addressed if the emerging obesity time bomb was to be defused. In 2001 the UK National Audit Office produced a major report on obesity[15] and this was quickly followed in 2003 by the Chief Medical Officer's report *The Obesity Time Bomb*.[16] Obesity as a key public health priority was now well established within government and it seemed that concerted government policy would now be applied to stop the increase.

Yet, despite all these reports linking food industry activities and poor food choices to obesity, government ministers refused to shift towards greater regulation. Ministers remained wedded to the approach of personal freedom and individual responsibility. But things were changing in Europe. In 1991 Sweden banned all television advertising directed at children under the age of 12 years. Restrictions on advertisements during children's programmes have been imposed in Greece, Norway, Denmark, Austria and the Netherlands.

In the UK a ban was introduced in January 2008 on advertisements for foods high in salt, sugar or fat during programmes whose viewers were mainly under the age of 16 years. This ban did not extend to programmes with audiences consisting mainly up of adults, even though many children watch them. Research from the Westminster Food and Nutrition Forum found that children were still seeing these advertisements and this was followed by calls for an all-out ban or the restriction of advertising to after the 9.00 p.m. watershed.[17]

Indeed, the limited effect of this partial ban had been foreseen by *Which?*, the consumer magazine, which predicted that advertisers, in response to the ban, would simply target television shows frequently watched by children.

The future

The continuing existence of significant inequalities in health between people in different social classes provides an indicator of the scale of population health improvements yet to be gained. Assuming that the environmental, social and economic advances made in the previous century can be sustained, a key issue for the future – as the 2004 White Paper *Choosing Health: Making healthy choices easier* emphasised – relates to the extent to which citizens will elect to use their wealth in ways that will help to reduce further not only the risk of premature death, but also of chronic illness in later life.[18]

Health promotion service or sickness service?

In the second half of the 20th century, 'public health' was focused on problems associated with increasing wealth: high consumption of tobacco and usually high-quality (but too often fatty and/or salty) foods, coupled with reduced physical activity levels. These challenges required new types of state, corporate and individual responses involving balancing the needs and rights of individuals, and supporting market freedoms, with the need for appropriate public leadership and regulation to assure health gains are preserved and, when and where possible, new ones are attained. The strategy must be to seek effective prevention and, when disease strikes, early treatment whenever possible and combine this with later-stage disease treatment or palliation whenever necessary. This effectively is the remit of a national health service.

Seen from this perspective, debates about whether or not the UK NHS is a 'health promoting service' as opposed to a 'sickness service' are arguably outdated. A more integrated approach to primary and secondary illness prevention and treatment needs to be developed, which addresses risk reduction and early diagnosis but does not lose sight of the legitimate needs of people with chronic disease. For such a service to work effectively, voluntary commitment from individuals and communities will need to be combined with appropriate regulatory intervention. Individuals, charities, companies and government must continue to work together to identify common goals and to use their combined resources to achieve them.

This was the vision of Derek Wanless when he came to assess long-term funding for the NHS.[19] In short, Wanless recommended a much greater investment in prevention of disease and particularly in ensuring that the population was 'fully engaged'. What this means is that each individual needs to reassess his or her personal responsibility for health to ensure that there are sufficient resources to go around. As Wanless has noted obesity is now, and will be in the next 20–50 years, the main driver for diseases that will have the potential to bankrupt the NHS as it is currently constituted.

Nutrition and health

A 'fully engaged' public will be difficult to bring about without concerted effort. When it comes to nutrition and the role it plays in health, the complexity can be staggering and creates huge challenges for governments attempting to deal with their populations. Emerging economies such as India and China, as a result of globalisation, are finding that parts of their populations are achieving rapid prosperity and as a result are exhibiting the same health problems associated with overconsumption of food at the same time as others in their population are malnourished.

Industrialisation of our societies and the associated lifestyle that wealth brings is at the root of our obesity problem. The political imperative for a government was, and largely still is, to feed its population and the easiest way to do this is, where possible, to leave food supply to the market. Politics and economics have always played a central role in human nutrition and it is this political and economic story that sets the backdrop for our current obesity epidemic. It is somewhat of an irony that our obesity problem is merely an unintended consequence of the politics of food.

Politics of food

Human health is inextricably linked to nutrition and this holds true at an individual, community and societal level. In the modern era, from the Industrial Revolution to the present, but in common with the whole of human history, the Nation's health can be measured by prevailing nutritional standards. In the past, poor food quality and insufficient available calories were to blame; famine was a frequent occurrence throughout human history, and in many parts of the world it remains so.

For nations such as Britain learning to cope with industrialisation, it was accepted that Malthusian economics ruled. This simple cause-and-effect economic model linked the size of a population to its ability to feed itself; the size of the population increased to the point where food supply was exhausted and then famine cut the population back.

The current obesity epidemic in developed nations has its origins in the food and other policies of the past 200 years but its direct causes are more recent; certainly there is a link to 1954, when post-war rationing ceased but also and more specifically to somewhere in the past 30 years. Despite the fact that body mass index has increased year on year since the early 1900s, a tipping point was reached sometime in the 1970s and once passed, the obesity problem emerged. It is unlikely that one or even a few factors are to blame. Many variables conspired together in a complex, chaotic fashion to create the national expanding waistline and a stable social system that will prove difficult to reverse.

Fat chance of staying thin

Clearly what an individual, a community or a social class eat is not the outcome of choices made of free will; choices are constrained by a wide range of factors such as the price of food, culture preferences, customs, ecological factors and international trade agreements. All these factors conspire to restrict and direct the individual's and the community's food choices.

The complexity of food politics reflects the complexity of global economics and the regulations associated with them. The politics of food and the way a nation feeds itself is closely linked to the market and how it operates. From the Industrial Revolution to the present day, the history of food in developed countries serves to provide some understanding of why many in the population are now, or are becoming, overweight or obese.

Our daily bread

During the Industrial Revolution, growing urban populations stimulated British landowners to increase agricultural production of wheat, while at the same time technical innovations, and the development of land for the specific purpose of growing wheat, led to an increase in production. Wheat replaced barley, rye and oatmeal that were, up to then, the staple food grains used in Britain. By 1760, 60% of the population consumed wheat-based bread, by 1820 this was up to 80% and by 1890 it had risen to 90% giving wheat dominance of the nutritional economy. For this key reason it became more expensive and difficult to purchase bread other than white bread made from wheat.[20]

The growth of the population was so great and the dominance of wheat so significant, that by the end of the 1700s Britain became a net importer of wheat. These imports supplied the nation's needs up to the time of the Napoleonic Wars when a blockade of Britain by France cut off imported wheat supplies and prices went up. This was good for English landlords who gained financially but not so good for the rest of the population, particularly the poor who, because of the dominance of wheat, were now dependent on bread for survival. The end of the Napoleonic Wars in 1815 saw the return of imported wheat but Parliament, in an effort to halt wheat importation that resulted in reduced price and reduced income for landowners (many of whom were Members of Parliament) enacted the Corn Laws which were only repealed fully in 1849 having been seen as a key stimulus in the creation the Irish Famine of 1846–1849.

Britain now depended more on affordable imported wheat and there was an increase in supply from the gigantic plains of the mid-west of America which were for the first time being crossed by railroads. In 1877 North American wheat imports to Britain stood at 2.5 million tonnes, approximately 40% of all the wheat consumed, and this significantly reduced the price of wheat by 50% between 1873 and 1893. By this time wheat bread had become firmly established as the bread of the poor as well as the rich but increasingly dominated the diet of the underprivileged.[21]

Technical innovations

The roller mill was first used in Britain in 1878. With steam power it allowed large-scale production of wheat flour. In addition the roller mill made it possible to separate the husk of the wheat grain and the wheat germ from the starchy endosperm. Now flour was white as the public desired; white bread, it was felt, had more flour in it. With the increasing use of technology, white bread was now available to the poor and as roller mills flourished the poor had little access to any other bread. Interestingly brown bread such as the Hovis loaf, introduced in 1892, was more sought after by the middle classes who ate it for its health qualities.

Commercial baking was at this time popular as it reduced the long and tedious chore of home-baking bread, and also saved fuel. In Manchester, for example, there were no commercial bakers in 1800 but by 1835 there were 650 to serve the tripling of the population.[20]

Milling and baking became dominated by a small number of very large producers able to introduce technologies and take advantage of economies of scale. In 1935 there were around 2000 millers but, by 1978, only two companies – Rank-Hovis-McDougall and Associated British Foods – accounted for 75% of milling output and 61% of all bread production. A key element in restricting food choices was already appearing.

Big Sugar

With the introduction of cheap sugar to Britain from the 1780s, following the development of sugar plantations in the West Indies, a cheap and important ingredient was now available for the British diet. Based on the slave trade, sugar plantations were worked by slaves transported from the west coast of Africa to the New World. The ships that ferried them returned to England laden with sugar and cotton.

Sugar had a number of attractive characteristics. It was good at preserving foods in jams and in condensed milks, popular with poorer families since they were highly palatable, cheap and were less perishable.

Sugar also formed the basis of the confectionary industry that was started in the mid-19th century by the famous Quaker families: Fry, Rowntree and Cadburys. It was a combination of cheap flour and sugar that formed the basis of the cake and biscuit industries. Indeed sugar is a very flexible and important component in making foods palatable and desirable, over and above its sweetness. It imparts a viscosity to the food, for example, tomato ketchup, and 'mouth feel' which is a key element in the popularity of carbonated drinks.[22]

Today Big Sugar, a pejorative term used to define the global sugar industry, can be divided into the sugar food industry – confectionary and biscuits – and the sugar water industry – soft drinks. The latter is dominated globally by two brands: Coca-Cola and Pepsi. Interestingly, both Coca-Cola and Pepsi were developed by pharmacists.

The contribution of the sugar water industry to the obesity crisis has only begun to be realised. The sugars in soft-drink products originally were mainly glucose (from cane sugar) but from the mid-1970s this changed to fructose when scientists in Japan found a way to produce a cheaper sweetener from corn syrup, termed high-fructose corn syrup (HFCS). This is six times sweeter than cane sugar and made from corn, which was in surplus supply at the time. HFCS meant that the cost of producing soft drinks could be slashed, and using it in frozen food protected the products against freezer burn. It was very flexible, providing longevity for products in vending machines and it conferred a more natural look to biscuit products.[22]

Soft drinks can be consumed easily and in large quantities and in many individuals, particularly the young, it becomes easy to consume excessive calories. There is less of an impact on the body's satiety system from soft drinks, so a larger number of calories can be consumed from sugar-based drinks than sugar-based foods.

Marketing and merchandising by the sugar water industry has always been innovative and has set international marketing standards. The presence of soft drinks vending machines in American and British schools – both junior and higher – was nothing short of a national scandal. Vending machines have been taken out of primary schools but the transition in secondary schools has been slower.

Industrialisation of food

Wheatgerm – a by-product of the roller mills – was turned into farm animal food and became the basis of the dairy industry. Food processing became important, and as it did so, the food manufacturing industry was increasingly concentrated in the hands of a small number of producers who exerted greater control over food retailing and, to some degree, farming.

Supermarkets and food labelling

Humans are pre-programmed genetically to take the easiest route possible – the route that expends the least resources. Difficult-to-obtain items are less likely to be used. The 'optimal default' theory dictates that, in any given scenario, the most obvious, natural or 'default' path to take ought to be that which is the healthiest.[23] According to the theory, a person entering a public building should be drawn to using the stairs rather than the lift. Ideally, cycling to work should be made an easier option than taking public or private transport. This would require dedicated cycle lanes, secure bicycle racks, and showering and changing facilities at work. Similarly in supermarkets, the most obvious option to choose ought to be the healthy one. 'Diet' products with low fat ought to be the norm, and high-fat options labelled as such: Diet Coke or Coke Zero should be easier to find on the shelf than the unhealthier version, which should be more expensive, hard to reach, and have ugly packaging. Although this seems difficult to imagine, given the commercial world in which we live, the optimal default is a concept that should merit better understanding from public health campaigners.

This is important because, in Britain, four supermarkets dominate the supply of foods and ultimately consumer choice. It is in this context of these deep-rooted and long-term trends in the UK agriculture, food and retail industries that our modern pattern of food consumption and health must be understood as it has set the basis for the current obesity epidemic.

Food labelling is an important element in helping consumers to shop and eat more healthily. Food labels should provide easily accessible and understandable information, which can be rapidly assimilated by a busy shopper who only has a few seconds available to choose any one particular brand. A product containing a massive 15% fat should not be misleadingly labelled 85% fat-free, and a low-fat product containing high levels of sugar should not be able to masquerade as a healthy product. Accurate and informative food labelling will only succeed as a weapon in the fight against obesity if the information and education required is already targeted towards consumers, in order for them to understand the complicated facts and figures involved in making the correct choice. As would be expected in such a complex arena, there is no easy way to pinpoint accurately the most effective method of labelling food, and different retail outlets have different stylistic outlooks.

Guideline daily amounts (GDAs) is a scheme being promoted by a number of the main supermarkets in the UK, yet the simpler and more effective Traffic Light System (TLS), advocated by the Food Standards Agency, works better and is being ignored by most supermarkets, Sainsbury's being one exception.

In a pilot in 2004, one of the big supermarket chains claimed that the TLS produced a 'positive response' from customers but their in-depth research 'highlighted deficiencies' and the supermarket chain abandoned the TLS in favour of GDA (T Tonks, Tesco's company nutritionist, personal communication, 2007). They found that sales of certain highly popular foods fell when the TLS was used – but this is exactly what needs to happen if we want to avoid digging bigger graves for people who will be dying younger. Customers exposed to the TLS were viewing the red-coloured food labels as a deterrent rather than a warning. One supermarket felt that this was inappropriate as these foods could be eaten, if not all the time. The company abandoned the TLS in favour of GDAs, which they use on the front of packaging on over 7000 foods.

The GDA scheme, unsurprisingly, does not reduce sales of unhealthy foods because it is too complex for people to understand when they are rushing through the food aisles. The GDA scheme provides information on the five nutrients – calories, fat, saturates, sugars and salt – and only provides a benchmark to set the grams per serving into context, but this is a time-consuming job and difficult for the average consumer, which is why most supermarkets prefer to use it.

The food industries too have been mostly against food labelling and much of the labelling regulation currently in operation has been forced on the industry when voluntary practices have not been adhered to. The preferred option for the Food Standards Agency is a common scheme across the UK that is easy to understand and allows consumers to glean sufficient information from the front of the packaging to make a healthy choice. Traffic lights would appear to be the obvious options: red indicates too much, green is good.

Sainsbury's, who have adopted the TLS scheme, have also noticed that certain foods became less popular where they had a red colour flashed on their packaging. Rather than see this in a negative way the company are committed to progressing the scheme and adjusting its product offering accordingly. It works in getting people to choose and, as a result to eat, healthier foods.

The fast-food industry

The fast-food industry started life in the US in the 1940s and slightly later in the UK and Europe, and it may hold a vital clue to the cause of our obesity epidemic. The obesity epidemic is often blamed on the reduction in physical activity in our work and leisure lives, but increased calorific intake is an equally important factor. Estimates of food intake too often rely on monitoring goods purchased in shops, and discounting food eaten outside the home. Somehow it seems too simplistic to charge one sector with all the blame yet the fast-food industry's rise has been parallel with an increase in the numbers in the population who are overweight and obese. This linear relationship is of course not an indicator of causality but it is an attractive proposition, and one that national governments are rightly becoming concerned about.

In the UK between 1984 and 1993 the number of fast-food outlets doubled at the same time as the prevalence of obesity doubled. Obesity is much less prevalent in Spain and Italy where spending on fast food is relatively low. There has not, however, been a clear-cut causal relationship between the expansion of the fast-food industry and the national waistline but the evidence is strong.

In China, the proportion of overweight teenagers has roughly tripled in the past decade. In Japan, eating hamburgers has, it is claimed, added to the rate of obesity. During the 1980s, the sale of fast food in Japan more than doubled and the rate of obesity among children soon doubled. Today one-third of all Japanese men in their thirties are overweight and associated diseases are increasing, not only in the indigenous population, but also in migrants outside Japan.[21]

In 2008 the Japanese government introduced mandatory 'fat checks' for the over-40s. This initiative is targeted at reducing the annual health costs – currently the equivalent of £1.5 billion – and might serve to increase the cost of medical insurance for those with an expanded waistline.

Japan has moved rapidly from a diet based around fish, rice and vegetables and including little red meat, dairy and processed foods towards a modern Western diet. Japanese men are faring worse than women: men are now 10% heavier then they were 10 years ago, whereas women's weight has increased by 6.4%.

The biggest problem is still in the USA. In 1970, Americans spent around $6 billion on fast food; in 2001 they spent more than $110 billion.[22] On any given day, 25% of the adult population visit a fast-food outlet. The social impact of the fast-food industry, initially in the US, then in the UK and Europe and more recently globally, has not only been to transform the diet but also to impact on the built urban environment, popular culture and even the social fabric of society. In essence, it might not have created the obesogenic environment but it certainly endorsed and concentrated it. It is this very same toxic environment that, through market forces, is being replicated globally.

The fast-food revolution of the past 50 years reflects the change in popular culture that has many more drivers. The car culture that developed in the US in the 1940s and 1950s was a stimulus towards a built environment designed around the car and an impediment to exercise. Furthermore, labour-saving devices in the home offered improved individual freedom and more leisure time.

In 1975 about one-third of American mothers with young children worked; today this figure is two-thirds. This has impacted on the way food is prepared. In the 1960s in the US, three-quarters of the money used to buy food was spent on food prepared in the home. In 2000 half of money used to buy food was spent in restaurants; mainly of the fast-food variety. About 90% of the spend on food in the US is on food that is processed.

The fast-food industry's success is based on a commitment to business principles: quality, efficiency, uniformity and marketing. This pursuit has produced successful global brands such as McDonald's, Burger King and Kentucky Fried Chicken. Customers are drawn to familiar brands by an instinct to avoid the unknown. Marketing is core to the success of fast-food brands and this was the first industry to apply marketing techniques directed at children. Among the marketing developments they created was marketing synergy, where products loved by children were linked to fast foods, for example, Disney characters to McDonald's Happy Meals. This ploy was hugely successful; through 'pester power' parents were forced to visit fast-food restaurants more regularly and, crucially, reliance on nostalgic childhood memories of a brand ensured lifelong loyalty. Most American schoolchildren could identify Ronald McDonald, a McDonald's character.[22] KFC, McDonald's and Coca-Cola are the most recognisable brands in the world. Coca-Cola is the favourite drink among Chinese children. McDonald's first opened in China in 1992; eating there raises a person's social status. Sadly, eating like the Americans is ensuring that other nations are beginning to take on the Americans' body morphology as well as their appetite.

Whereas the foods served in fast-food restaurants seem familiar, they have been completely re-formulated over the past 40 years as the industry has improved its efficiency. The food it produces, resulting in significantly reduced costs, meant that working class families in the 1970s could, for the first time, afford to feed their children in restaurants. Now, for the first time, this is starting to happen in Chinese cities.

The taste of fast-food fries is largely determined by the cooking oil used. From the 1960s into the 1990s, McDonald's cooked french fries in a mixture of 7% cottonseed oil and 93% beef tallow, giving the fries the unique and much sought-after taste. This also gave the fries more saturated fat per gram than a McDonald's hamburger.[21] In response to intense criticism, this changed in the 1990s, with a switch to pure vegetable oil enhanced with 'natural flavours' to ensure taste consistency.

Processed foods are given their proper taste by a flavourist who will also consider issues such as a food's 'mouth feel' – the unique combination of textures and chemical interactions that affect how the flavour is perceived. Mouth feel is modified by the use of fats, gums, starches, emulsifiers and stabilisers. A french fry's crispness, for example, is determined by the process of rheology, involving the treatment of starches in the potatoes to ensure that they do not stick in the manufacturing process. In the autumn, sugars are added to the potatoes, whereas in the spring, sugar is leached out, maintaining the uniformity of taste throughout the year.

In the US cattle are fed on corn to ensure rapid fattening and tender meat, enhanced by anabolic steroids that restrict the supply of American beef to Europe. The feedlots of the US were a success following World War II. The meat of grain-fed beef is fatty and tender unlike grass-fed beef, which required ageing for a few weeks before consumption. Grain-fed beef is ready for eating a few days after slaughter. Chickens bred for the fast-food industry are highly processed and have a fatty acid profile that more closely resembles beef than poultry, as they are cooked in beef tallow. Chicken nuggets contain twice as much fat per gram than a hamburger.

As people eat more meals outside the home, they consume more calories, less fibre and more fat. Over the past 40 years the per capita consumption of carbonated soft drinks has quadrupled. In the 1950s a soft drink in a fast-food restaurant contained about 8 ounces (224 g); today a child-size drink is 12 ounces (336 g) and a large Coke is 32 ounces (896 g) – approximately 310 kcal.

In 1972, McDonald's added large fries to its menu, and these were 'super sized' in 1992. Super-size fries have 610 kcal and 29 g of fat. A taste for fat developed in childhood is difficult to lose as an adult.

Conclusion

The complex relationship between nutrition, exercise, politics and health is articulated in the Whitehead and Dahlgren model (figure 4.1). In industrialised nations, and some sectors of developing nations, the environment in which individuals live has, as a result of powerful market forces, become obesogenic. Many factors conspire to reduce the activity levels and more frequent eating of calorie-dense foods. Owing to the complexity involved, it proves difficult to address the problem and government policy is often compromised, accommodating vested interests such as the food lobby. In addition, the information that needs to be provided to the public, such as through effective food labelling is often not provided in a way that people can easily use, especially in making healthy choices. Addressing the obesity epidemic will require a concerted effort at all stages of the Whitehead and Dahlgren model.

References

1. Open University U205 Course Team. *Health and Disease: Health of Nations.* Milton Keynes: Open University Press, 1985.
2. Chief Medical Officer. Annual Report. *Health Check – On the State of the Public's Health.* London: The Stationery Office, 2002.
3. Olshansky S *et al.* A potential decline in life expectancy in the United States of America in the 21st Century. *N Engl J Med* 2005; 352: 1138–1142.
4. Dahlgren G, Whitehead M. *Policies and Strategies to Promote Social Equity in Health.* Stockholm, Sweden: Institute for Futures Studies, 1991.
5. Whitehead M, Dahlgren G. *Concepts and Principles for Tackling Social Inequalities in Health. Studies on social and economic determinants of population health,* No. 2. Copenhagen, Denmark: WHO Regional Office for Europe, 2006.
6. Erkki V *et al.* Cardiovascular risk factor change in Finland 1972–1997. *Int J Epidemol* 2000; 79: 449–450.
7. Lawrence J. Confusion of public health message. *The Independent,* 8 May 2008.
8. Sugar Association (USA). *WHO Report on Diet, Nutrition and Prevention Misguided.* Washington DC: Sugar Association, 2003.
9. Offer A. Body weight and self-control in the United States and Britain since the 1950s. *Soc Hist Med* 2001; 14: 79–106.
10. Royal College of Physicians. *Storing Up Problems: the medical case for a slimmer nation.* London: RCP, 2004.
11. Rose G. *The Strategy of Preventive Medicine.* Oxford: Oxford University Press, 1992.
12. *The Black Report and The North South Divide: Inequalities in Health.* London: Penguin, 1992.
13. Scottish Intercolligiate Guidelines Network. *Management of Obesity in Children and Young People.* No 69. Edinburh: SIGN, 2003.
14. World Health Organization/Food & Agricultural Organization. *Diet, Nutrition and the Prevention of Chronic Diseases.* WHO Technical Report Series 916. Geneva: WHO/FAO, 2003.
15. National Audit Office. *Tackling Obesity in England.* London: The Stationery Office, 2001.
16. Chief Medical Officer. *The Obesity Time Bomb.* London: The Stationery Office, 2006.
17. Westminister Food and Nutrition Forum. *Food Labelling Policy. Nutrition and Food Science,* 38, 2008.
18. Department of Health. *Choosing Health: making healthier choices easier.* London: Department of Health, 2004.
19. Wanless D. *Securing Good Health for the Whole Population.* London: HM Treasury, 2004.
20. Barasi M, Mottram R F. *Human Nutrition,* 4th Edition. London: Edward Arnold, 1987.
21. Schlosser E. *Fast Food Nation.* London: Penguin, 2002.
22. Critser G. *Fat Land.* London: Penguin Books, 2003.

5

Metabolic basis

In times of plentiful nutrition, in common with much of animal kingdom, humans store energy by laying down fat in adipose tissue and building up glycogen stores in the liver. This ensures an energy source in leaner times, conditions often encountered when humans roamed the African savannah a million years ago. Natural selection favoured humans who were metabolically energy efficient and the storage of calories in adipose tissue was an important aspect of this. In prehistoric times, our hunter-gatherer ancestors spent most of their time crossing the savannah in search of food that was never in ample supply.[1]

To ensure that humans were highly focused on obtaining food, natural selection favoured a human brain that was highly motivated – 'hard-wired' – to seek out energy-rich foods, particularly fats and simple sugars. A ripe fruit tree was a prized find and early humans were highly motivated to search for them. Likewise, huge effort was expended in seeking out sources of fat, mainly from animals killed by other, more efficient predators, such as lions or cheetahs or killed by human hunters themselves. Since humans were not as fast or as efficient as other mammalian hunters in the savannah, there was a need to be social in hunting and this sociability extended to the sharing of food among the hunters and within the group so that females with babies were supported. By eating communal meals, the group bonded and was more successful, and individuals were more likely to survive, reproduce and raise the helpless infants. Lacking technology, early humans would not have been capable of storing food for use at a later time. Foods are highly perishable so storage in the body was the only option and the human body evolved for this purpose.[2]

Humans are designed metabolically for a life on the savannah, a highly active existence where high-energy foods were normally in short supply and were supplemented by less energy-rich foods such as roots and tubers. In the modern world, our efficient metabolism becomes a problem. We now live in an environment where easy access to high-energy, inexpensive foods is assured with little, if any, energy needed in obtaining them. Our efficient metabolism, which allowed us to survive lean times, is now causing us to store excessive amounts of energy mainly as fat and this is a significant risk to our health. Furthermore, in our various cultures, we have retained the nurturing and socialising roles associated with the food that we eat – food is part of our social interaction. A mother instinctively feeds her children and her love is often reflected in this feeding role. Socially food is important. The communal meal is now the lunch with friends, the dinner with family or business colleagues.

We also eat food, however, for two metabolic reasons: to provide fuel for energy and to obtain the building blocks for new body structures. Fuel and building blocks are provided from three basic molecular food groups: carbohydrates, proteins and fat. In addition, vitamins and minerals are provided in food and act as the 'tools' by which metabolism proceeds efficiently.

In this chapter we consider the metabolic basis of nutrition, to provide a background to our understanding of what constitutes a healthy diet – a diet that provides sufficient energy and nutrients. Debate rages, particularly within the fad-diet industry, on the most effective weight-loss diet. Since the 1950s, based on the work of Ansel Keyes[3] and then supported by national nutritional policy such as the McGovern report[4], low-fat diets were deemed more healthy than low-carbohydrate diets. It was assumed that high-fat diets led to individuals becoming overweight and obese but, more importantly, caused disease, which was the main focus of Ansel Keyes's work.

This view has been challenged in recent years particularly through the popularity of high-fat, low-carbohydrate diets such as the Atkins Diet (see Chapter 7, pp. 114 and Chapter 13, pp. 224). Proponents of high-fat, low-carbohydrate diets suggest that the focus on low fat within national nutritional policy was incorrect. On the contrary, they argue, it is carbohydrates that are the main reason for the explosion in the numbers who now suffer from obesity. In short, carbohydrate stimulates insulin production and this is the reason for the increase in obesity and type 2 diabetes. So is it a 'low-fat, high-carb' or a 'high-fat, low-carb' diet that is best? An understanding of human metabolism – an appreciation of the fundamentals of how the human body derives its energy from foods consumed – will give a better insight into the current arguments that are proving difficult for the lay person to understand fully. What we choose to eat will impact significantly on our metabolism and can affect the degree of weight gain or weight loss experienced. That said, it is clear that irrespective of whether 'high-fat, low-carb' or 'low-fat, high-carb' is shown to be right in the end, the average individual in the UK and the US is consuming more calories than are needed for day-to-day metabolic needs and it is this more than anything that is the source of the current obesity epidemic.[5]

Carbohydrates

Carbohydrates are a family of compounds consisting solely of carbon, hydrogen and oxygen. The elements are arranged in six carbon rings, strung together in chains and on this basis carbohydrates are termed simple (few rings) or complex (many rings). This is an important distinction as it determines the role of specific carbohydrates in metabolism. The simple carbohydrates are the sugars and contain one or two rings (monosaccharides and disaccharides) – essentially they are sweet to taste. Complex carbohydrates are long-chain polysaccharides and can be divided, depending on how the chains are hooked, into starches that are digestible (starch and glycogen) and fibre (an indigestible form).

Sucrose (table sugar) consists of one molecule of glucose linked to one molecule of fructose. Maltose consists of two glucose molecules. Lactose, the milk sugar, consists of one molecule of glucose linked to one molecule of galactose. Starches composed of perhaps thousands of linked glucose molecules are the most common digestible polysaccharide.[6]

Glucose, galactose, sucrose, fructose, maltose and lactose are simple sugars and the body can convert these directly into energy or they can be turned into fats. Glucose, galactose and fructose are monosaccharides (one-ring). The disaccharides are sucrose, maltose and lactose. Both polysaccharides and disaccharides are digested in the gut and converted into monosaccharides, mainly glucose, before being converted to energy within cells or stored as glycogen or fats (figure 5.1).

Glycogen consists of many hundreds of glucose units linked together. Glycogen is an efficient form in which to store glucose; it is insoluble and therefore does not exert an osmotic pressure, it has a higher energy level than the corresponding weight of glucose, and it is easily broken down by enzymes into glucose under the influence of the hormone glucagon. About 10% of the mass of the liver and 1% of our muscle consists of a glycogen. It is compact, highly branched and stored in the form of small granules about one to four thousandths of a millimetre across.

Insulin in carbohydrate metabolism

Insulin is a hormone secreted by the pancreas in response to a rise in blood glucose following a meal. It is primarily responsible for glucose homeostasis stimulating the build up of glycogen in the liver from glucose, and facilitating the metabolism of glucose for energy, effectively reducing the blood glucose concentration. In addition, insulin is also responsible for the conversion of amino acids to proteins and fatty acids to triglycerides.

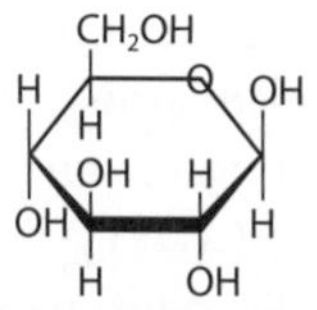

Figure 5.1 Chemical structure of monosaccharides.

During food deprivation, in non-diabetic individuals, the liver becomes the body's main source of available carbohydrate. In this circumstance a low blood glucose concentration results in a low plasma concentration of insulin and enzymes in the liver are stimulated to produce glucose (gluconeogenesis) as a source of energy. Low blood sugar levels trigger the formation of two hormones in the pancreas, glucagon and adrenaline, that stimulate the break up of glycogen stores into glucose.

When food is again eaten, and consequently blood glucose is elevated, insulin is again secreted and insulin feedback to the liver will switch off gluconeogenesis.

In diabetic patients there is insufficient insulin, or none at all; therefore, gluconeogenesis proceeds out of control. Large amounts of glucose are produced but cannot be utilised for energy or converted to glycogen owing to the lack of insulin necessary for the processes. Fats and proteins are broken down to provide the liver with an alternative energy source. Eventually the glucose concentration in the blood exceeds the ability of the kidneys to re-absorb it after glomerular filtration and therefore glucose appears in the urine (glycosuria).

High levels of glucose in the urine create an osmotic effect, which depletes the body of water, resulting in large quantities of urine being produced (polyuria) and consequently severe thirst (polydipsia).[7]

During gluconeogenesis there is excessive release of fatty acids into the circulation, which are used as an alternative source of energy. An enzyme cleaves a two-carbon moiety off a fatty acid molecule to produce acetyl-co-enzyme A (acetyl-CoA). The latter is used to produce ketone bodies such as acetoacetate, acetone and betahydroxybutyrate, which are used as a substitute for glucose. Unfortunately these ketone bodies cannot be metabolised fully and their presence causes metabolic problems. In uncontrolled diabetes mellitus, the blood stream is swamped with glucose and ketone bodies; eventually these overcome the blood buffering system and the plasma pH falls, resulting in diabetic ketoacidosis which can be rapidly fatal.

Energy in ATP

Glucose is the body's main source of energy as its combustion in cells drives the formation of the energy-rich molecule adenosine triphosphate (ATP). ATP is the energy that powers all cellular processes. Approximately 40% of the energy derived from the metabolism of food is conserved in ATP molecules. ATP represents a coiled spring; the three phosphate groups each possess a negative charge. Splitting off one phosphate group by hydrolysis produces adenosine diphosphate (ADP) releasing the energy inherent in the repelling negative charges of the phosphate groups. This process can be repeated with the loss of a second phosphate group with subsequent release of energy, producing adenosine monophosphate (AMP).

Cycles

Burning sugar is a two-stage process. Firstly, glucose undergoes glycolysis by a sequence of 10 enzyme-catalysed steps to pyruvate, and ATP molecules are consumed in the initial phase of this process, producing ADP. The result of the complete conversion to pyruvate is a total gain of two ATP molecules for each glucose molecule consumed.

Pyruvate then enters the second stage of combustion; the citric acid cycle, a stage that requires oxygen. When oxygen is unavailable this stage can occur anaerobically and pyruvate is converted to lactate. Sudden vigorous exercise such as a sprint will occur anaerobically but this is not sustainable for very long and a build up of lactate is associated with cramp. Aerobic metabolism is relatively inefficient and extreme exercise leads quite quickly to muscle fatigue; energy is consumed faster than it can be produced.

The citric acid cycle utilising oxygen is more sustainable. The process is conducted in the mitochondria. In the mitochondrion, pyruvate is enzymatically converted to acetyl CoA. Fatty acids and glycerides from fat metabolism also generate acetyl CoA.

In simple terms, the citric acid cycle produces electrons used to convert oxygen and hydrogen ions into water. This process releases energy and it is this energy that is captured for the production of ATP molecules.

Fats and cholesterol

Fat is the general term used for a range of chemical compounds that are insoluble in water and are metabolised in the body. The triglycerides are the most important fats and are composed of one molecule of glycerol and three molecules of fatty acid. Fatty acids vary in the size of their carbon chain, ranging from as few as four to as many as 20. In addition to the variable lengths, fatty acids also differ in the number of hydrogen atoms per carbon atom. Palmitic acid has 16 carbons and no double bonds and is known as a saturated fatty acid – it has the maximum possible number of hydrogen atoms and is normally solid at room temperature, certainly on refrigeration. Oleic, linoleic and linolenic acids each have 18 carbons and two oxygen molecules but they differ in the number of double bonds; oleic has one double bond (monounsaturated), linoleic has two and linolenic has three (polyunsaturated). Fatty acids that are unsaturated, either polyunsaturated or monounsaturated, will be liquid at room temperature.

Linoleic acid is an essential fatty acid since it cannot be produced intracellularly in humans, and must be derived from food. Plant-based foods are generally a good source of polyunsaturated fatty acids (the exception being palm oil and coconut oil). Seafood is rich in monounsaturated and poly-unsaturated fatty acids.

Omega-3 fatty acids – the main polyunsaturated fatty acid in many fish oils – is first unsaturated at the third carbon from the 'omega' end in the fatty acid chain (the end with three hydrogens). Eicosapentanoic acid is one of the chief omega-3-fatty acids in fish oil. In contrast, omega-6 fatty acids such as linoleic acid are found in plants; a rich source is oil of evening primrose.

Compound lipids are formed from fatty acids, glycerol and various nitrogen-containing bases and often contain phosphate groups. They are integral parts of the general cell structure and phospholipids are, for example, an important group of compound lipids.

Cholesterol

Cholesterol is not a fat but, like fats, it is insoluble in water. It is a vital body component used as a building block for cell membranes and certain steroid hormone molecules. Cholesterol's insolubility has required the body to develop an ingenious means to transport it in the circulation and it does this in conjunction with other fats, proteins and phospholipids.

Cholesterol is transported in microscopic bodies called lipoproteins (figure 5.2). Total serum cholesterol accounts for all the cholesterol distrib-uted among these lipoproteins, either as free cholesterol or as esters.

There are four main types of lipoproteins, which are classified according to their densities. Each contains differing amounts of cholesterol, triglyc-erides, phospholipids and protein (figure 5.3).

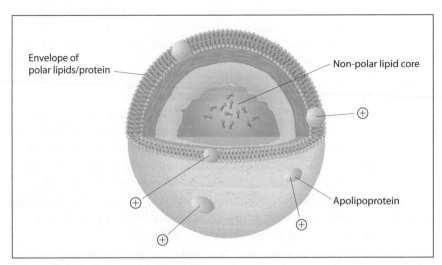

Figure 5.2 Chemical structure of lipoprotein.

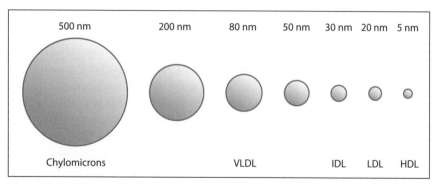

Figure 5.3 Relative size/density of the main lipoproteins in the circulation.

Low-density lipoproteins (LDLs) contain the highest amount of cholesterol (46%). The other lipoproteins are very low-density lipoproteins (VLDLs), high-density lipoproteins (HDLs) and chylomicrons.

Another means of describing lipoproteins is by their apoprotein type a component of the outer wall of the lipoprotein. Each lipoprotein has a specific apoprotein attached – LDLs have an apoprotein B100 – and these proteins assist removal of lipoproteins from the circulation when they are attached to liver receptors (see figure 5.4).

The surface of liver cells contain specific receptors for apoproteins, and a deficiency in the number of receptors or a genetic defect in their structure means that removal of lipoproteins from the circulation is reduced, leading to accumulation of cholesterol in the blood stream and ultimately deposition on to the walls of arteries (atherosclerosis).

The transport mechanism for cholesterol and other dietary fats in blood was first established by Brown and Goldstein in the early 1980s.[8] Chylomicrons are formed in the intestine as a result of digestion and taken up into

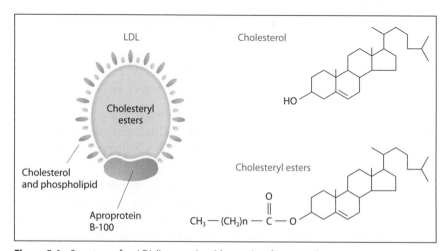

Figure 5.4 Structure of an LDL lipoprotein with associated apoprotein.

the blood stream, transporting dietary triglycerides and cholesterol from the gut to the liver.

While in transit from the gut to the liver, chylomicrons come into contact with the enzyme lipoprotein lipase, found on the surface of capillary endothelial cells. This enzyme removes some of the triglyceride content, leaving a chylomicron remnant. The chylomicron remnants reach the liver and are absorbed into the liver cells. The liver synthesises VLDLs and excretes them into the circulation. When in the circulation they come into contact with lipoprotein lipase, which removes triglycerides, leading to the formation of LDLs. LDL is the major supplier of cholesterol to peripheral tissue. Individuals with a higher ratio of LDL to HDL have a higher risk of coronary heart disease. HDL is also synthesised in the liver, and in the circulation it transports free cholesterol back to the liver where it can be secreted as free cholesterol or bile salts into bile. Since it removes cholesterol, having high levels of HDL lessens the risk of coronary heart disease.

Fats are derived from a range of foods and this is covered in Chapter 11.

Fat from food

With little, if any, fat metabolism occurring in the stomach, most fat digestion occurs in the small intestine. The predominant enzyme is pancreatic lipase working in association with bile that acts as an emulsifier and essential element in the process. Fat is incompletely digested in the duodenum, producing a combination of glycerol, fatty acids, disaccharides and mono-saccharides.

Utilisation of fats

After absorption, fat is dealt with in three main ways:

- oxidation to provide energy
- storage as triglycerides
- used as components for the building of tissue structures.

Oxidation of fat involves metabolic dissimilation of fat; a piece of the fat molecule – the active acetate – is cleaved off and becomes an intermediate to the production of high-energy phosphate ATP which makes the energy inherent in fat available to the body.

Fat, unlike carbohydrate, may be stored in the body in large amounts and on average forms over 10% of body weight. This is equivalent to 7 kg in an adult, representing some 7000 kcal of food energy, or more than one month's total food reserve. In people who are overweight the fat reserve is much greater.

Triglycerides are not deposited interstitially between cells or fibres. Rather they are taken up by adipose cells, which in effect become an envelope for a large fat droplet. Adipose tissue therefore selectively absorbs triglyceride fat, mostly saturated fat when it is available (in times when food is plentiful) and releases fat when needed (in times of starvation). The activity of adipose tissue is under hormonal control and is key to the development of obesity.

The triglycerides in adipose tissue are derived from two main sources in food: fat and carbohydrates. Fat released from adipose tissue is rapidly taken up by the liver and broken down by hydrolysis into glycerol and fatty acids by the liver enzyme lipase. Glycerol is utilised by carbohydrate metabolism. The fatty acids are oxidised to acetyl CoA, each containing two carbons, and these fragments are either metabolised completely to CO_2 and H_2O with energy liberalisation or recombine to give acetoacetic acid – a four-carbon moiety, a ketone body by a process of ketogenesis, and if unchecked resulting in ketosis. Ketogenesis is the process that is rampant in poorly controlled diabetes and is discussed above in the section on insulin. In this situation, owing to the lack of insulin, there is an inability to produce energy from glucose. The liver then increases metabolism of fat.

Fatty liver occurs where the liver contains massive deposits of neutral fat, and is the result of a high-fat diet.

Glucose to fat

Dietary carbohydrate (glucose) can be converted into fat because the pathway of carbohydrate and fat metabolism meet at the common intermediate acetyl-CoA. Since fatty acids are reversibly formed from acetyl-CoA this means transformation of carbohydrate via pyruvic acid and acetic acid into fatty acids is possible. Indeed this transformation is promoted by insulin and depressed by anterior pituitary hormone. Alternatively fats are hydrolysed to glycerol and converted into triose and join the main pathway for carbohydrate metabolism (figure 5.5).

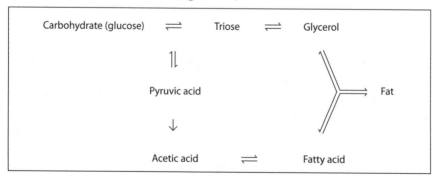

Figure 5.5 Metabolic conversion of glucose to fat.

Conversion of fat to carbohydrate is an extremely inefficient process with only 12 g of blood glucose provided from 100 g of fat.

Fat as a source of energy

Fat is an important direct energy source providing 9 kilocalories per gram (kcal/g), compared with 4 kcal/g for carbohydrate and protein. Triacylglycerol, whether in the form of chylomicrons or other lipoproteins, is not taken up directly by any tissue, but must be hydrolysed outside the cell to fatty acids and glycerol, which can then enter the cell.

Lipolysis (fat breakdown) and beta-oxidation occurs in the mitochondria. It is a cyclical process, in which two carbons are removed from the fatty acid per cycle in the form of acetyl-CoA, which proceeds through the Krebs cycle to produce ATP, CO_2, and water.

The main sites of triglyceride synthesis are in the liver, adipose tissue, and intestinal mucosa. The fatty acids are derived from the hydrolysis of fats, as well as from the synthesis of acetyl-CoA through the oxidation of fats, glucose, and some amino acids. Lipogenesis from acetyl-CoA also occurs in steps of two carbon atoms.

Carbohydrate is converted to triglycerides, using glycerol phosphate and acetyl-CoA obtained from glycolysis. Ketogenic amino acids, which are metabolised to acetyl-CoA, may be used for the synthesis of triglycerides. The fatty acids cannot fully prevent protein breakdown, because only the glycerol portion of the triglycerides can contribute to gluconeogenesis.

Most of the major tissues (e.g., muscle, liver, kidney) are able to convert glucose, fatty acids and amino acids to acetyl-CoA. However, brain and nervous tissue – in the fed state and in the early stages of starvation – depend almost exclusively on glucose. Not all tissues obtain the major part of their ATP requirements from the Krebs cycle. Red blood cells, tissues of the eye, and the kidney medulla gain most of their energy from the anaerobic conversion of glucose to lactate.

Storage of fat

Fat is stored in adipocytes and to some degree genetic factors determine an individual's fat distribution pattern. This pattern is largely governed by the regional activity of the enzyme lipoprotein lipase. This enzyme is responsible for the uptake and storage of fat in adipocytes. In addition to being responsible for inter-individual variation in fat distribution, it is also responsible for changes in fat distribution in pregnancy and in middle-age as well as explaining why black people have less visceral fat than whites. The gender distribution of fat is also explained by regional activity of lipoprotein lipase;

adipocytes in the hips, thighs and breasts produce considerable LPL activity in females, whereas abdominal adipocytes show the greatest LPL activity in males. This explains the 'apple' and 'pear' shapes characteristic of males and females respectively.[9]

Obesity results from an increase in the numbers of adipocyte cells and in the size of the adipocytes. Obese people have perhaps three times more cells and their cells are 50% larger than non-obese individuals. In explaining the cellular difference between obese and non-obese individuals, it is adipocyte cell numbers rather that cell mass that counts.

An average-size person (75 kg) has between 25 and 30 billion adipocytes and the average lipid content of each adipocyte is 0.6 μg. The clinically obese individual has three to five times this number of adipocytes, particularly when the obesity occurs in childhood and in adolescence.

A classic study in 1971[9] followed a number of obese adults as they reduced body weight by an average of 46 kg (149–103 kg). Before the weight reduction the average number of adipocytes was 75 billion (they were obese patients) and after the weight reduction this number remained the same. The weight loss was achieved by a 33% reduction in size of the adipocytes from 0.9 μg of lipid per cell to 0.6 μg of lipid per cell.

When this group achieved a normal body weight of 75 kg by losing an additional 28 kg, adipocyte numbers remained the same, whereas cell size continued to shrink to 0.2 μg per cell. This size is much less than the size of an adipocyte in a normal weight individual (who has never been obese). What seems to be happening is that in obese adults there is no means of reducing the number of adipocytes, only their size, and consequently the individual is more prone to regaining weight.

A number of studies, also in the 1970s, considered the effect of weight gain on adipocytes and these support this idea of cell size rather than cell number being of key importance.[9] Individuals, all adults, were fed high-energy diets and over time this increased their body weight by 25%. Adipocytes increased in size but not in number, so what is clear is that overeating in adults resulting in moderate increase in weight increases the size of existing adipocytes but does not increase the number of fat cells.

However, where energy intake is excessive and causes adipocytes to enlarge to their upper limit of about 1.0 μg fat per cell, then additional cells are produced from the pre-adipose pool. In addition, the liver is stimulated to take up more fat and fat is also stored between muscle fibres. In adults, therefore, it is difficult to increase fat cell numbers yet this is very different in children. A significant increase in the number of fat cells has been shown to occur at key stages in childhood development, particularly during adolescent growth spurts. In many ways this research suggests that the core of a national obesity problem stems from nutritional habits that stimulate increases in fat cells number in early life, and since these cell numbers are not reduced over time it become increasingly difficult to reduce body mass in adulthood.

Bottle feeding and the early introduction of solid food is associated with childhood obesity. Breastfeeding on the other hand allows the infant's natural appetite to set limits on food intake and delaying the introduction of solid foods may prevent overfeeding, development of poor eating habits and subsequent obesity.

Targeting children and young adults with programmes that increase physical activity and calorie restriction can reduce body fat. Because cell size not cell number decreases, it is vital early on in life to ensure that children's diets avoid filling the existing adipocytes as this cellular pressure stimulates the proliferation of cell numbers that make keeping weight down in adulthood very difficult.

Cellulite

For purposes of completion and because it is so widely discussed in contemporary culture, it is worth considering cellulite. Cellulite is a controversial condition as it is a construct of the cosmetic industry rather than a medical issue; the term 'cellulite' is not listed in medical dictionaries. The fat layer within the skin is located in the subcutaneous layer of tissue called the hypodermis. The thickness of the fat layer, which varies greatly from one person to another, depends on the size and number of fat cells.

Everyone, whether old or young, curvaceous or slim, has fat cells under their skin. Cellulite occurs as these fat cells swell and the surrounding fibrous tissue changes in texture, causing a pulling effect and giving the skin a dimpled look. Hormonal changes also contribute to cellulite, which partly explains why women are more prone to it, and genes are thought to play a part. Cellulite appears largely on the thighs and bottom, but can be found on the inner knees, hips, lower abdomen and under the arms.

In short cellulite is likely to benefit from a moderate loss of weight but it is unlikely, in the absence of weight loss, that it can be improved by application of creams and ointments.

Proteins

Proteins are the building blocks of the body but also, particularly in times of starvation, they are a source of energy. Throughout the plant and animal kingdoms there exists an astonishing array of proteins, all composed of different variations of 20 amino acids. Amino acids are composed of acetic acid, an amino group (NH_2) with a carbon spine that is variable in length.

The general formula for an amino acid is $R.CHNH_2.COOH$ where R refers to various short chains of carbon rings, with hydrogen, oxygen,

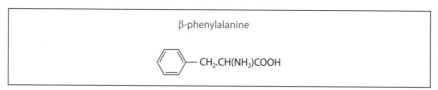

β-phenylalanine

CH₂.CH(NH₂)COOH

Figure 5.6 Chemical structure of phenylalanine.

sulphur or even further NH_2 groups. Figure 5.6, for example, shows the structure of the amino acid phenylalanine.

When amino acids are linked to form proteins, they do so through the NH_2 group of one amino acid reacting with the COOH of another amino acid, splitting off water in the process as it creates a peptide link. Proteins can be hugely complex fragile structures and their activity in the body is dependent on the maintenance of this structure.

Digestion

Because of the complexity of proteins, a single peptidase enzyme cannot split up a protein chain into its constituent amino acids in the way that glucosidase or lipase can split polysaccharides or fat into glucose or fatty acids respectively. Several different peptidases act on the proteins, each specific for a peptide bond with a particular side-chain on the amino acid. Other enzymes attack each end of the peptide chain, lopping off single amino acids one after another.

In the stomach, pepsin works on the protein in food and this enzyme works best in an acid environment. The pancreas secretes another three enzymes: trypsin, chymotrypsin and aminopeptidase. The combination of the effects of these three enzymes digests proteins to single amino acids which are absorbed into the blood. The majority of amino acids pass to the liver and are absorbed into the liver cells (hepatocytes) and some will pass to other tissues from the main circulation.

Protein as a source of energy

In the liver cells, in the absence of glucose or fats, amino acids will be converted by enzymes into a source of energy. Deaminases remove the amino portion and change the molecule into urea, which is subsequently excreted. After the amino group has been removed the residual is changed either to glucose or to fatty acid, depending on the amino acid involved. Leucine, phenylalanine and tyrosine are changed to fatty acids and then to acetic acid. Alanine, glutamic acid and other amino acids are change to glucose. The fatty acid and glucose can then be used as a source of energy. About 60% of protein follows the glucose pathway and the rest the fatty acid path.

Where carbohydrates or fats do not accompany protein intake, amino acids will not pass the liver but will be used as a source of energy for the body. Where fat or carbohydrate is present in the food, these act as inhibitors of deaminases, the amino acid escape their action, pass into the general circulation and can be used for tissue-building purposes.

There is a constant interchange between the amino acids of the circulation and those of the tissues. Some amino acids are used to make creatinine essential in carbohydrate metabolism in muscle. In starvation, tissue-based amino acids will be used to provide energy. In these situations, amino acids are turned to glucose. For this reason, starvation diets achieve part of their success by reducing the body's lean tissues. It is this lean tissue that provides the key to glucose metabolism and its initial removal makes further weight loss more difficult.

Exercise has a profound effect on muscle growth, which can occur only if muscle protein synthesis exceeds muscle protein breakdown; there must be a positive muscle protein balance. Resistance exercise improves muscle protein balance, but, in the absence of food intake, the balance remains negative. The response of muscle protein metabolism to a resistance exercise bout lasts for 24–48 hours; thus, the interaction between protein metabolism and any meals consumed in this period will determine the impact of the diet on muscle build up. Amino acid availability is an important regulator of muscle protein metabolism. The interaction of post-exercise metabolic processes and increased amino acid availability maximizes the stimulation of muscle protein synthesis and results in even greater muscle build up than when dietary amino acids are not present.

Hormones, especially insulin and testosterone, have important roles as regulators of muscle protein synthesis and muscle cell hypertrophy. Following exercise, insulin has only a permissive role in muscle protein synthesis, but it appears to inhibit the increase in muscle protein breakdown. Ingestion of only small amounts of amino acids, combined with carbohydrates, can transiently increase muscle protein anabolism, but it has yet to be determined if these transient responses translate into an appreciable increase in muscle mass over a prolonged training period.

References

1. Leakey R. *The Making of Mankind*. London: Book Club Associates, 1981.
2. Winston R. *The Human Mind*. London: BBC, 2003.
3. Keyes A, ed. Coronary heart disease in seven countries. *Circulation* 1970; 41 (Suppl): 1–211.
4. McGovern Report. *Dietary Goals for the United States*. US Senate Select Committee on Nutrition and Human Needs, 1977.
5. Taubes G. What if it's all been a big fat lie? *New York Times Magazine*, 7 Jul 2002.
6. Barasi M, Mottram R. *Human Nutrition*, 4th edn. London: Edward Arnold, 1987.

7. Woteki C, Thomas P. *Eat for Life. The Food and Nutrition Board's guide to reducing your risk of chronic disease.* Washington DC: National Academy Press, 1992.
8. Brown M S, Goldstein J L. A receptor-mediated pathway for cholesterol homeostasis. *Science* 1986; 232: 34–47.
9. Hirsch J. Adipose cellularity in relation to human obesity. In: Stollerman G H, ed. *Advances in Internal Medicine*, vol. 17. Chicago: Mosby Year Book, 1971.

6

Hunger, appetite and satiety

Human beings need nutrients to survive and since the process that allows us to obtain these nutrients, eating, is an essential yet voluntary activity (unlike breathing and the beating of the heart), Nature has ensured that eating, like having sex, is something that we desire, even crave, and therefore it is something we are 'hard-wired' to do. Hunger is the body's signal that we need food and our appetite ensures that we consume sufficient amounts of calories and other nutrients, where sufficient might be defined as enough to satisfy immediate needs and then some more for future use. When we have eaten sufficiently, satiety signals kick in and we stop eating. The 'gut–brain–adipose axis' is central to the control of feeding behaviour and metabolism. Satiety is a major factor in the control of meal sizes and this mental perception is produced by neural, endocrine and nutritional inputs during meal ingestion.[1]

Evolutionary pressures therefore have selected out those humans for whom the seeking of highly nutritious and energy rich foods was a priority. These individuals were more likely to survive and reproduce, passing on genes for survival in an environment where highly nutritious foods were uncommon. The human brain is genetically programmed to prioritise the search for food and it is further programmed that when food is obtained, the individual is motivated to eat sufficient to cover current metabolic needs and to eat some more because, in the environment in which early humans lived, it might have been some time before the opportunity to eat again arose.[2] Clearly, in Western and other evolving economies of the world, this is no longer the case – indeed, it is very often the opposite.

Physiological factors

Human physiology, as a result of genetic selection pressure, is precisely engineered for a very different environment to the one we find ourselves living in today: our obesogenic environment. A man will consume approximately 900 000 kcal per year yet, even in today's obesogenic environment, there is normally only a balance of about 11 kcal per day, resulting in the average person putting on a few pounds in weight each year (there are

3500 kcal in one pound (imperial) of fat). So despite our concerns about obesity and its medical consequences, it is surprising that the problem, given our environment, is not much worse than it already is. So how can human physiology maintain with such precision the necessary energy balance?

What has evolved in humans is a hugely complex physiological feedback system, most of which has only been identified in recent years, with much more still to be uncovered. One of the most important factors, in physiological terms, is that satiety is a weak signal, whereas hunger is a strong signal. For this reason, a lack of symmetry in this aspect of our physiology, humans are more likely to respond to hunger signals and to eat than they are to respond to satiety signals and stop eating. Physiologically we are designed to get fat.

A variety of psychological and physiological factors interact to regulate feeding behaviour. The hunger–satiety cycle involves pre-absorptive and post-absorptive humoral and neuronal mechanisms interacting in a highly complex fashion. These signals are primarily designed to stimulate eating and conserve energy when adiposity levels are low, rather than inhibiting eating and expending energy when adiposity increases. In this way it is an asymmetrical system and not a very effective feedback process, although studies have shown how deliberately overfed young – but not older – volunteers return spontaneously to their normal body weights over several months.[3]

Clearly, as the obesity epidemic shows no sign of abating, the human body has found ways of overcoming the strong physiological control of weight, and the weak satiety signals, and this has happened for various reasons. Genetic factors go some way to explaining who does and does not gain weight, and how much, neatly demonstrated by overfeeding studies in twins.[4] Statistical analyses have demonstrated that possibly 50% of the variation in body mass index between individuals has a genetic basis but that these effects are mainly polygenic influences, affecting appetite behaviour, spontaneous physical activity and basal metabolic rate, and that hundreds of genes are jointly responsible. But genetic factors alone cannot explain the current epidemic – our genes have not changed much in the 30 years since obesity started becoming a serious public health issue.[5] Increasingly sedentary lifestyles take their toll; a lumberjack burnt off at least 5000 kcal per day, the average modern male only half that amount, but food intake has not reduced accordingly. More than 50 years ago Morris and colleagues[6] famously demonstrated that vigorous physical activity was crucial to cardiovascular fitness, and the lack of such activity helps override the precise regulation of weight.

Intrinsic regulation of food intake is also easily overcome by increases in the energy density of food, for example, high-fat suppers that allow no compensatory adjustments until the following morning.[7] Furthermore, sugary drinks in particular circumvent meal-based regulation of appetite. Consumables with greater energy density, rich in fats, refined sugars, and starches, are thoughtlessly consumed in greater amounts, based on their palatability, rather than their nutritional status. The urge to eat sugary and salty foods is driven by selective taste buds and neuronal projections to the limbic pleasure centres, and the combination of the fats and sugars, rare and precious in our early evolution, is especially alluring.[8]

The science of appetite regulation, especially with regard to obesity, is complicated and far from being comprehensively understood. The brain has a continuous conversation, or dialogue, with the gut, so that the brain can govern the amount of food eaten, compared with the amount required by the body.[9] The brain receives messages from all five senses via the cerebellum: the sight of a sumptuous feast, the sound of bacon sizzling, the smell of garlic from the kitchen, the feel of food being prepared, and of course the taste of a favourite dish. Just like Pavlov's dogs, who salivated at the sound of the dinner bell, these sensations induce the desire to eat, as the brain sends messages through the autonomic nervous system telling the stomach to prepare itself.[10]

The gut also has ways of communicating to the brain that it needs food, indicating the time to go hunting. Messages to and from the gut travel via the autonomic nervous system, leading to increased activity of the gut muscles, increasing peristalsis, borborygmi (rumbling), and hunger pangs, and by way of hormones released from the gut, which stimulate hunger and increase food intake, such as ghrelin.

In response to all these heightened sensations, we eat. The gut then contacts the brain in different ways – the nerve endings in the stomach wall transmit impulses directly via the vagal nerve, to inform it that food has arrived. In addition, with increasing amounts of food entering the bowel, the cells of the gut produce a number of hormones (PYY_{3-36}, obestatin, cholecystokinin), which are released into the blood stream and circulate around the body. These hormones are monitored by the brain stem, and the hypothalamus, which respond by producing messenger chemicals called neuropeptides (NPY, AgRP) that give us the sensation of being satisfied, and full, so we should stop eating.

The desire to eat, and the sensation of hunger, however, are distinct, and different phenomena, and it is possible to override the effects of these chemicals, so that we can eat when we are not actually hungry, because of the external cues that make eating enjoyable. These sensations are governed by brain neurotransmitters, which control eating behaviour, the most important being serotonin, which is the target for one of only two available anti-obesity drugs. However, the endocannabinoid system has recently been discovered, the blockage of which alters eating behaviour, inducing weight loss.[10]

Once a person has become overweight or obese, the dialogue between the gut and the brain is joined by a third party: fat. Far from being merely an inert mass, adipose tissue is one of the most active glands in the body, but unlike other glands, such as the liver or thyroid, which are beneficial, fatty tissue is highly toxic. It produces chemicals called cytokines, such as tumour necrosis factor-α, and interleukin-6, which cause inflammation, particularly in the lining of the blood vessels, leading to heart disease, and in other organs such as the liver. Adipose tissue also secretes a hormone called leptin, the function of which is to tell the brain how much energy is stored in the body, hence obese people have high levels of leptin, but may be resistant to its action.

Strong and weak signals

Signals that govern eating can be broken down into a number of behaviours that appear to be discrete:

- meal initiation
- maintenance of eating (intra-meal controls)
- meal ending (satiation, and inter-meal satiety).

Meal initiation

Psychological, social and environmental factors coupled with food availability, metabolic processes and gastric contraction result in the origin of hunger signals that brings about the eating behaviour.

In adapting to our environment, humans use an external clock to control daily routines, particularly sleeping and eating. Lunchtime, for example, is a psychological trigger that stimulates an individual to experience hunger. This is hunger as a learned behaviour and is not created by a fall in body calories. Smell, taste and texture of food also trigger hunger, yet these aspects are culturally learned and are personal preferences. For example, where an individual does not like curry, the smell of curry will not trigger hunger. Interestingly, people will feel hungry for a particular taste: sweet, sour, bitter and salty, and this even extends to colours. Looking at a yellow banana can stimulate the desire to eat; a red banana would not do the same thing. Similarly, the sight of red or green can trigger hunger (the desire to eat) for an apple, but this will not happen if the apple is blue. So in response to our senses (smell, sight, feel) our brains are stimulated and create a desire to eat.

Ghrelin, the hunger hormone, appears to be key to the stimulation of hunger and is hypothesised to be the main factor leading to meal initiation. Discovered in 1999, our understanding of ghrelin and its role in appetite and eating behaviour is only in its early stages.[11] The hormone is released from the stomach and its release can be brought about by a number of factors, such as habit and the sight and smell of food. Daily habit, such as the time we take lunch, is also an important trigger for ghrelin release. Studies have shown that where an individual normally eats a meal at 8.00 a.m., 1.00 p.m. and 7.00 p.m., these times are associated with a blood ghrelin spike at or just before these times; therefore it seems that our internal daily clocks programme us to feel hungry at specific times when food is expected. Studies have confirmed that if a snack is introduced at, say, 3.00 p.m. and this snack is maintained as part of the daily routine, in a short time this will result in a blood ghrelin spike at 3.00 p.m. and a resultant feeling of hunger. Conversely, where a meal is dropped from the daily schedule for only a few days, the blood ghrelin spike is diminished and hunger is no longer experienced at this time.

Since ghrelin is so important in stimulating the sensation of hunger, it is postulated that gastric surgery might not only be successful because of a reduced capacity for food but also because ghrelin spikes are reduced, leading to a diminished feeling of hunger across the day.

Ghrelin released from the gut into the blood is effective in stimulating a number of brain centres: the hindbrain (responsible for automatic and subconscious processes), the mesolimbic system in the midbrain (responsible for pleasure and desire) and the hypothalamus (governs metabolism).

Interestingly in patients with anorexia, rather than having a deficiency in ghrelin, as would be expected, such individuals are found to have chronically high ghrelin levels, but in this psychiatric condition the hunger response is ignored and overridden.

Ghrelin might also provide a common brain pathway to explain the mechanism behind patients who overeat and become obese as well as patients with a drug addiction. In both groups there is a lack of activity for ghrelin in the mesolimbic system within the brain, and it is postulated that overeating or taking mood-enhancing drugs might be a means of attempting to stimulate this brain region and obtaining the desired pleasure effect.[12]

Ghrelin's access to the brain is through the melancortin 4 receptors (MC4-R). These act as a neural gateway for the hormone and where a mutation of MC4-R exist this might explain either an overactivity or underactivity of brain response and thus obesity could, for some with altered receptors, be described as a genetic disease.[12]

Food craving

Our moods and our emotions affect our eating patterns and vice versa. Whereas the relation between food and mood is poorly understood, there is an emerging body of research linking eating and mental state. Mood can have a significant influence on the decision when to eat and what to eat. The *serotonin theory* first put forward in the 1970s suggests that consumption of carbohydrates alters the balance of amino acids in the blood, which in turn results in increased brain serotonin.[13] Serotonin is a mood enhancer and, therefore, to improve mood, individuals crave and seek out food rich in carbohydrate. As recently as the late 1980s, others[14] suggested that carbohydrate might even reduce depression, since there is some link to seasonal affective disorder and premenstrual syndrome: those affected have low mood and apparently seek out carbohydrate foods. Yet there is little evidence to support the serotonin theory, since only when the content of a meal has less than 2% protein will blood amino acid levels favour a rise in serotonin. Very few meals will achieve this, even foods that are supposedly high in carbohydrates such as potatoes and bread.[15]

Additionally, there is little evidence that foods such as chocolate or ice cream are craved for their carbohydrate content. They have a sweet taste but have a higher fat content. It is more likely that chocolate is craved not for its sugar, fat or psychoactive content but because of its sensory effect in the mouth. Indeed a classic study[16] seems to prove that chocolate craving is due to sensory factors, rather than the presence of pharmacologically active substances. Participants with a chocolate craving were given a series of boxes containing milk chocolate, white chocolate, cocoa powder capsules or white chocolate with cocoa. Each of these products contained similar concentrations of psychoactive agents and calories. When they experienced a chocolate craving they opened a box and ate the contents. Only milk chocolate satisfied the cravings and it was concluded that the sensory pleasure in the mouth was the main reason why people chose chocolate.

Maintenance of eating

Once a meal is started, factors controlling the meal size are soon initiated but with some delay to allow for the maintenance of appetite, so that sufficient food can be consumed. Because of the delay between the swallowing of food and the digestion of food, the satiety mechanism requires a short-term signal to prevent overeating. This short-term satiety signal, cholecystokinin, is activated by psychological factors, chemical senses (taste and smell) and mechanical factors, mainly processes of swallowing and gastric distension. Long-term satiety is activated by the chemical sensing of nutrients and peptides in the gastrointestinal tract, by the liver and in the brain.[17]

The *boundary theory* of hunger[18] suggests a significant cognitive aspect to hunger. It suggests that there are boundary lines between hunger and satiety and these are determined biologically. The space between those two boundaries is controlled cognitively, in other words, people decide how much they think they should eat, and if one sets a satiety boundary cognitively lower (for example, during a weight-reduction diet) than one that is biologically predetermined, the body tries to compensate food intake to meet the biologically determined boundary level by triggering hunger. For the obese, this biologically determined satiety boundary is higher than for the non-obese.

Set-point theory[19] seems to be a more recent version of the boundary theory and suggests that for an individual, his or her weight is predetermined and set by the hypothalamus. Once set, the body attempts metabolically to maintain that weight. This theory suggests reduced-calorie diets do not work because of a specific set-point weight. In patients who are obese, the fault lies in the set point being too high, owing to damage to the ventromedial hypothalamus.

Some evidence to support these theories exist. In a study on a US university campus, students were invited to taste ice cream samples. They were told that the purpose of the experiment was to determine their taste preferences. Participants were grouped into dieters – individuals who frequently dieted – and non-dieters – individuals who did not normally restrict calorie intake by diet. They were each given very large portions of ice cream for the taste trial – more than would normally or practically be needed for a tasting test. Results from the study showed that dieters, those who were constantly going on calorie-controlled diets, consumed a much greater amount of the ice cream sample than non-dieters. It was concluded that, since dieters were more likely to be cognitively controlling their portion intake when given permission to eat – as they thought they were in this taste test – they were more likely to eat more, as they depended on a cognitive, rather than a physiological, process to tell them when they had eaten enough. Non-dieters were less dependent on a cognitive process to control portion size and were more sensitive to satiety signals.[20]

In a second study,[21] researchers measured the number of crackers eaten by subjects over a period of time, as the real time was manipulated by a faster or slower clock. They showed that obese people are more affected by the clock time than the real time. Obese people respond to external cues of hunger, such as time, more than non-obese people, who respond more to internal cues of hunger. These studies provide some good evidence for the cognitive influences on the amount an individual will eat and thus the impact on the prevalence of obesity.

Endocannabinoid system

It has been known for years that those who used cannabis as a recreational drug often over-ate while under its influence. The 'munchies', as it is known to cannabis users, was better understood with the discovery of the endo-cannabinoid system, a endogenous hormonal system that has a role in the maintenance of eating once a meal is started and a key role in central and peripheral regulation of energy balance and fat accumulation. The drug rimonabant (Acomplia) blocks this system and thus supports weight loss but the suspension of its marketing authorisation in October 2008, because of an increase in psychiatric problems, including suicide and suicide ideation, underpins the complexity of the brain processes generally as well as those involved in hunger and satiety.[22]

The endocannabinoid is of course an endogenous system with its own endogenous ligands – anandamide and 2-arachidonylglycerol – and the receptors CB_1 and CB_2 are produced in response to certain stimuli such as hunger, as well as the smell, taste or texture of food. Cannabis users merely hijack these receptors using the external ligand δ-9-tetrahydrocannabinoid to elicit the positive feelings associated with cannabis use. When activated, the ligands interact with the receptors and increase the intake of food and accumulation of fat. The ligands, produced from phospholipid precursors, have a very short half-life being quickly degraded by metabolism once they have achieved their effect. The CB_1 receptor is associated with eating, whereas CB_2 is related to the immune system and may be irrelevant in terms of obesity. CB_1 receptors are widely distributed around the body and can be found in the brain, muscles, liver, gastrointestinal tract and the pancreas. In simple terms, when an individual is hungry, there is a massive rise in brain levels of these ligands. Following the consumption of food the levels of these ligands fall. The endocannabinoid system is known to be overactive in obese subjects, in contrast to its dormant status in normal-weight individuals.

The means by which these ligands create their effect is complex, and is a process known as 'retrograde suppression of neurotransmitter release'. In simple terms, the impact of CB_1 receptor stimulation in the synapse is to prolong the effect of GABA (γ-aminobutyric acid) which leads to prolonged eating. Blocking of the receptors, such as with the rimonabant, leads to weight reduction.

Meal ending

Cholecystokinin

The satiety neuropeptide cholecystokinin, a peptide hormone secreted in the duodenum, is responsible for stimulating the digestion of fat and protein by causing the release of pancreatic digestive enzymes and bile. It also acts as a hunger suppressant.

In this way cholecystokinin plays a central role in the management of hunger and satiety – a role first identified when researchers were studying its effect on the gut. Subjects given doses of cholecystokinin do not want to eat, regardless of how much time has elapsed since their last meal. Receptors for cholecystokinin exist in the spleen, the gut and in the brain and thus it is a key messenger in the gut–brain axis that controls hunger and satiety. Following a meal, as the fat content is moving through the gastrointestinal tract towards the gallbladder, cholecystokinin is released, which promotes a feeling of satiety through a signal received in the brain. At this time cholecystokinin also signals the gallbladder to release bile, promoting the digestion of the fat and this also enhances the feeling of fullness. Other foods can also have this effect – potatoes, with no fat content, are reported to contain the proteinase inhibitor II (PI2), which promotes the release of cholecystokinin.[23]

Cholecystokinin is relatively short lived and does not act alone but interacts with several other hormonal signals, which in combination control eating. The other signals include amylin, oestradiol, glucagon-like-hormone, leptin and insulin. Amylin is synthesised by the pancreatic beta-cells and co-secreted with insulin and functions as a hormone to control satiety. Gastric load and the physical distension of the gut also plays a part in development of satiety.[24] It has been shown that eating is further decreased when cholecystokinin and the other signals were applied simultaneously, compared with cholecystokinin applied on its own.

Insulin and leptin appear to act by increasing the sensitivity of the brain to cholecystokinin. In this way, as food is consumed, insulin and leptin are secreted and, through their role in enhancing brain receptor sensitivity to cholecystokinin, there is an increase in the satiation signal and eating stops. Therefore, the integration of these messages within the brain – mainly in the hypothalamus – contributes to the sensation of satiation.

Leptin

The hormone leptin is produced by the adipocytes (fat cells). As the amount of fat stored in adipocytes rises, leptin is released into the blood and crosses the blood brain barrier, where it signals the hypothalamus directly that the body has had enough to eat. It also contributes to satiety by increasing the brain sensitivity to cholecystokinin.[23]

It is, however, a paradox that overweight and obese people, have high rather than having low blood leptin levels, suggesting that it is not just an increased blood concentration of leptin which supports a normal body weight but its impact in the brain. In obese individuals, what might be happening is that leptin is having difficulty entering the brain. The melanocortin-4 receptor (MC4-R) is one of the receptors that facilitate the movement of leptin across the blood-brain barrier and its ultimate entry in to the brain. Genetic errors in the MC4-R receptor, or possibly other blood-brain barrier gateway receptors, could explain why some individuals are more susceptible to obesity than others. About 10% of obese individuals show genetic mutations in the gene that regulates this compound. Developing an MC4-R agonist such as α-melanocyte-stimulating hormone (α-MSH) may affect how the central nervous system regulates adiposity.[25]

Alternatively, in obese individuals, there may be a failure of the interaction of leptin with other molecules such as cholecystokinin, which also affects feelings of satiety. It is likely that a network of chemical signals contributes to weight homeostasis and as yet some of these chemical messengers may not have been identified.

One of leptin's main effects may be to inhibit the synthesis and release in the hypothalamus of Neuropeptide Y, which increases food intake, decreases thermogenesis, and increases levels of insulin and corticosteroid in the plasma; however, leptin may have other targets and pathways both inside and outside the brain. A particularly important effect may be to suppress ingestion of fat without affecting carbohydrate ingestion.[26]

Genetics

Obesity is known to run in families, thus it has always been suspected to have a genetic basis. Analysis of the distribution of fatness in families suggests that a few major genes may act on a polygenic and environmental background, but it remains unclear which genes are involved; yet an obesity phenotype is highly likely to result from the interaction between an individual's genotype and his or her environment. Studies show that twins who grew up apart still weigh approximately the same, and adopted children's weights are similar to their biological parents, not their adopted parents.[27]

However, there is often the confounding factor of lifestyle, habits and diet. Twins and adoption studies have supported a substantial genetic influence on body mass index, with childhood environment having little effect. Various metabolic factors are known to be associated with the inherited tendency to be overweight, such as the single-gene defect resulting in obesity that includes Prader-Willi syndrome and Laurence-Moon-Biedl syndrome. However, single gene mutations, including the leptin-receptor mutation causing obesity, are rare and have little to do with the current obesity epidemic. In a way this is analogous to the rare occurrence of familial hypercholesterolaemia, which has little to do with the public health impact, in the general population, of raised serum cholesterol levels that were mainly the result of environmental factors.

Large babies only become fat adolescents when the father or the mother is overweight. If a normal-weight child under 10 years has one obese parent then the child's risk of becoming an obese adult is doubled. An individual's genetic make up does not necessarily cause obesity but it does lower the threshold for its development because of the impact of susceptible genes. However, a complete understanding of the role of genes, their mutations and the proteins that they create, in the accumulation of body fat and energy imbalance will require further research.[28]

Obesity therefore can have a genetic basis but it is most likely polygenic, with small variables contributing an increased risk of obesity in certain individuals. Such mechanisms have been described involving leptin and neuropeptides, such as proopiomelanocortin, neuropeptide Y, and the melanocyte-concentrating hormone receptors. The MC4-R receptor is acted upon centrally by proopiomelanocortin and α-MSH, both of which act to reduce dietary intake. Some investigators have suggested that mutations in the MC4-R gene can lead to increased proopiomelanocortin production and may be the single genetic cause of obesity.[29]

FTO gene

A genome-wide search for genes associated with susceptibility to type 2 diabetes identified a common variant in the FTO gene that predisposes to diabetes through an effect on body mass index. An additive association of the variant with BMI was replicated in 13 cohorts with 38 759 participants. The 16% of adults who are homozygous for the risk allele weighed about 3 kg more and had a 1.67-fold increased risk of obesity when compared with those not inheriting a risk allele. This association was observed from age 7 years upward and reflects a 15% increase in body fat.[30]

The FTO protein resembles enzymes that produce the penicillin antibiotics in bacteria and others that enable humans to sense and respond to changes in oxygen levels – for instance, at high altitude. FTO is most closely related to the AlkB family of enzymes, which, in bacteria, repairs DNA damaged by chemicals. The FTO protein can carry out this repair role and is targeted at the cell nucleus, as expected for a protein that modifies DNA. It seems that an obesity gene is having a direct effect on the FTO gene, which is turned on in regions of the brain concerned with appetite regulation, and that FTO levels decrease following fasting. Why or how can chemical changes to our DNA cause an increase in fat mass? As yet this is unknown but this will be a fruitful area of research in coming years.

What is known is that small variations in the FTO gene, which sits on chromosome 16, are more common among obese subjects. People with two altered copies of the gene were 3 kg heavier, on average, than those with normal copies. Only 35% of the white European population studied had two normal copies of the gene. Among adults, one-sixth of the population carries a 70% higher risk of being obese as a result of carrying variants in the FTO gene. In children the FTO gene may affect weight from as young as 7 years old.[30]

The mechanism of action of the FTO gene is unknown so it may be some time before the genetic basis of obesity is fully elucidated, yet it is unlikely that obese individuals can use a genetic excuse for abandoning good nutritional behaviour and increasing, then maintaining physical exercise.

References

1. Winston R. *The Human Mind and How to Make the Most of It*. London: Bantam Press, 2003.
2. Greenfield S. *Brain Story: unlocking our inner world of emotions, memories, ideas and desires*. London: BBC, 2000.
3. Roberts, S *et al*. Control of food intake in older men. *JAMA* 1994; 272: 1601–1606.
4. Bouchard C *et al*. The response to long-term overfeeding in identical twins. *New Engl J Med* 1990; 322: 1477–1482.
5. Allison, D *et al*. Genetic and environmental influences on obesity. In: Bendich A, Deckelbaum R (eds). *Primary Prevention Nutrition*. Totowa, NJ: Humana Press, 2001: 147–164.
6. Morris J *et al*. Coronary heart disease and physical activity of work. *Lancet* 1953; 2(6796): 1053–1057.
7. Morris J *et al*. Vigorous exercise in leisure-time and the incidence of coronary heart disease. *Lancet* 1973; 1(7799): 333–339.
8. Cotton J *et al*. Fat substitution and food intake: effect of replacing fat with sucrose polyester at lunch or evening meals. *Br J Nutr* 1996; 75: 545–556.
9. Raben A *et al*. Sucrose compared with artificial sweeteners: different effects on ad libitum food intake and body weight after 10 week supplementation in overweight subjects. *Am J Clin Nutr* 2002; 76: 721–729.
10. Haslam D, James W. Obesity. *Lancet* 2005; 366: 1197–1209.
11. McArdle W *et al*, eds. *Exercise Physiology: Energy, Nutrition and Human Performance*. Section 6. New York: Lippincott Williams & Wilkins, 2006: 844.
12. Del Guidice E *et al*. Molecular screening of the proopiomelanocortin (POMC) gene in Italian obese childen: report of three new mutations. *Int J Obes Relat Metab Disord* 2001; 25: 61–67.
13. Fernstrom J, Wurtman R. Serum serotonin content increase following ingestion of carbohydrate diet. *Science* 1971; 17: 1023–1025.
14. Wurtman R, Wutman J. Carbohydrates and depression. *Scientific American* 1989; 250: 68–75.
15. Benson D, Donoheo R. The effect of nutrition on mood. *Public Health Nutr* 1999; 2: 403–409.
16. Michener W *et al*. Pharmacological versus sensory factors in the satisfaction of chocolate craving. *Physiol Behav* 1994; 56: 419–422.
17. De Krom M *et al*. Common genetic variations in CCK, leptin and leptin receptor genes are associated with specific eating patterns. *Diabetes* 2007; 56: 276–280.
18. Herman C *et al*. Anxiety, hunger and eating behaviour: A boundry model analysis. *J Abnorm Psychol* 1987; 96: 264–269.
19. Keesy L, Powley B. Hypothalmic regulation of body weight. *Am Sci* 1975; 63: 558–565.
20. Schachter S, Rodin J. *Obese Humans and Rats*. Hilldale, NJ: Erlbaum, 1974.
21. Schachter S. *Emotion, Obesity and Crime*. New York: Academic Press, 1971.
22. DiMarzo V *et al*. Leptin regulated endocannabinoids are involved in maintaining food intake. *Nature* 2001; 410: 822–825.
23. Morgan, T, Bi S. Hyperphagia and obesity in OLETF rats lacking CCK-1 receptor. *Philos Trans R Soc Lond B Biol Sci* 2006; 361: 1211–1218.
24. Oesch S *et al*. Effect of gastric distension prior to eating on food intake and feeling of satiety in humans. *Physiol Behav* 2006; 87: 903–910.
25. Heymsfield S B *et al*. Recombinant leptin for weight loss in obese and lean adults: a randomized, controlled, dose-escalation trial. *JAMA* 1999; 282: 1568–1575.
26. Flier J, Spiegleman B. Adipogensis and obesity: rounding out the big picture. *Cell* 1996; 87: 377–389.
27. Eckhardt R. Genetic research and nutritional individuality. *J Nutr* 2001; 131: 131S–136S.
28. North M A. Advances in molecular genetics of obesity. *Curr Opin Genet Dev* 1999; 9: 283–288.

29. Wu P *et al.* Mechanism responsible for inactivation of skeletal muscle pyruvate dehydrogenase complex in starvation and diabetes. *Diabetes* 1999; 48: 1593–1596.
30. Frayling T *et al.* A common variant of the FTO gene is associated with BMI and predisposes to childhood and adult obesity. *Science* 2007; 316: 889–894.

PART 2

Towards management

This section considers approaches to the management of obesity and examines evidence of their effectiveness.

7

Prevention and interventions

Weight loss in primary care is only of interest as a method of improving a person's health, rather than his or her appearance, and is a means of modifying the cardiometabolic risk of those in the highest categories. For such individuals, a weight-loss target may be set at around 5–10%, a level which, when achieved by lifestyle intervention, has been shown to reduce progression to diabetes by an impressive 58% over 4–6 years.[1,2] The degree of weight loss achieved by some of the practice-based services is comparable to that induced in clinical studies and it should be remembered that a single unit decrease in body mass index (BMI) is associated with a reduction in incidence of type 2 diabetes by 13%.[3] Many other clinical benefits result, including reductions in cardiovascular disease risk factors, blood pressure and lipid profile.[4,5]

Weight management services must be focused on a reduction in the new incidence of obesity, as well as a reduction in the current prevalence in the population. A strategy that relies entirely on obesity prevention is futile; if no one from the normal-weight population became obese, thanks to a successful prevention strategy, there would still be epidemics of diabetes, heart disease and ultimately premature death over the coming decades, as already-obese individuals progress through the stages of illness. The only valid reason to prevent obesity is to prevent the subsequent co-morbidities; therefore an obesity prevention strategy is actually a diabetes and heart disease prevention strategy done on the cheap, because it ignores those at highest risk of diabetes and heart disease, i.e. those who are currently obese.

Current UK and European strategies such as the Foresight Report published in 2007[6] are guilty of glossing over the management of obesity, but obesity management must be prioritised alongside prevention for progress to be made. In recent years, a number of properly evaluated primary care services have appeared in the literature and this assessment would suggest that resources should be made available to support their roll out so that a greater percentage of the population might have access to and benefit from them.

At this time, however, as the evidence base evolves, public health is only starting to understand what a community-based weight management service might look like. This chapter examines the developing public-health-based approach to supporting those already overweight or obese, and helping them lose weight, and the more general population-approach, aimed at stopping normal-weight individuals becoming overweight or obese in the future.

Public health campaigns

Government has for many years issued public health information to ensure that the public have appropriate information on which to make lifestyle choices. This has not always been successful and often is down to the subtlety and the context of the information offered and the way this information is communicated. The public responded very differently to two public health campaigns in the 1980s. One featured the dangers of eating more than two eggs per day linked to increased risk of heart disease. The campaign had little impact on overall egg consumption, yet a news report about egg consumption carrying a risk of *Salmonella typhi* infection almost destroyed the UK egg industry. The difference in response was due to the perceived personal risk: an immediate, acute risk of vomiting and diarrhoea alters behaviour, whereas a non-acute risk, in the distant future, of heart attack or stroke is less effective in altering behaviour. Humans do not normally change behaviour when faced with a possible outcome that is years ahead.

In the 1980s, Scotland's health boards ran a hard-hitting anti-smoking television campaign featuring a young man with legs amputated as a result of smoking. It failed to get across the stop-smoking message, since the public simply did not believe the advertisement, as in the case of not eating more than two eggs per week. Assessment of this campaign suggested that the public did not trust government sufficiently, were aware of other public information messages that had in the past turned out to be incorrect or false, and had no personal experience of anyone in their thirties who had had a limb amputated due to smoking. As a result, current government health campaigns employ the same approach that any commercial organisation would adopt in public campaigns: they use focus groups. It is not easy condensing important yet complex health information and packaging it in such a way as to motivate the public to pick it up, internalise it and use it in their decisions about behaviour.

'Five-a-day'

The 'five-a-day' fruit and vegetable campaign has been largely successful, in that it has been widely adopted, although there are limitations in the way that the information has been interpreted, not least that 'five' is a completely arbitrary number which should be regarded as minimum intake; seven or ten would be better. Furthermore, some people fail to appreciate that potatoes are not included and, by logical extension, that chips are not one of their five-a-day. Indeed some commercial companies have been manipulating the message to sell 'fruit juice' that is so high in sugar content that they constitute a risk to health rather than a benefit. Others find difficult to decide what a 'portion' is. (A portion of fruit or vegetables is 80 g or what can be held in, and fill, an adult hand; one apple, pear, banana etc.)

Notwithstanding these concerns, there has been a greater uptake of fruit and vegetables in the UK diet as a result of this national campaign and the appreciation that the message must be kept simple will be key to the success of other public health strategies.

Public engagement

The UK government, especially through its four departments of health and also through other agencies such as local councils, has acted to address the wider determinants of health and to engage with communities and individuals in an attempt to ensure better understanding of good health and its link to a nutritious and balanced diet and to an increase in physical activity. Many primary care trusts in England, for example, are producing nutritional and activity initiatives targeted at local communities and individuals at high risk of becoming obese. A large amount of funding, about £30 million, was made available at the end of 2008 to support local authorities in creating more parks and cycle paths to make it easier for residents to keep fit. In addition, and as part of the same coordinated initiative, in late 2008, primary care trusts issued plans that were rolled out across England in 2008 and 2009 which included, for example, defining and creating walks and treks of varying distance and challenge, and supporting individuals to use these facilities. In Wales, some interesting initiatives, such as free-of-charge swimming for under-16s and over-60s are being funded by local health authorities. Whereas swimming on its own will not address obesity, it can serve to increase activity in those who dislike other forms of exercise and result in more active individuals. Groups such as Sustrans, which has a 'Living Streets' campaign, and the Active Travel Consortium are campaigning for safer streets for pedestrians, and better cycle routes. Natural England has many initiatives, including the Green Gym, whereby volunteers gain physical activity by restoring dry stone-walls and clearing overgrown gardens and orchards and other environmental projects. In this way changes to the local environment can support improvement in exercise – a key element in normalising body weight.

Change4Life

As part of the Change4Life campaign, hard-hitting advertisements showing the danger of fat gathering around internal organs in a £275 million government anti-obesity campaign were screened in December 2008.[7] Interestingly consumer research commissioned by the Department of Health for England as part of this initiative found that the public perceive obesity as a vanity problem rather than a health problem. In addition, a high percentage of the population do not regard foods such as cakes, biscuits, burgers, chips and crisps as unhealthy. This is logical given their cultural status and the wide availability of these products. However, this research did find that the idea of fat building up around internal organs has been associated with a high level of disgust and for this reason this feature was chosen as the target of the campaign.

The Change4Life campaign has the support of 34 commercial companies, many of which are normally associated with the manufacture and promotion of foods that are unhealthy. In addition these companies are also providing funding for the advertising campaign. A further aspect of the campaign is that a few supermarkets have agreed to reduce the price of fruit and vegetables whereas another company is funding breakfast clubs in deprived areas to ensure that children eat what is the most important meal of the day.

The Change4Life campaign therefore is a unique and exciting collaboration between central government, local health authorities and the food industry and, whereas this is to be applauded, it will be interesting to see how it works. It is much too early yet to see the benefits of the initiative. It may be that Change4Life becomes a watershed where commercial food companies, who until recently were opposed to any initiative that might have the potential to damage their market share, have now realised their role in obesity and as a result their social responsibility. Other commentators[7] have suggested that this alliance is only a means by which the food industry, which has been under intense political pressure to do something about the role their foods play in obesity, 'use this as a means of kowtowing to government and pushing up sales'.

Obesity management services

Clearly the most effective solution would be the provision of a wide range of initiatives that are attractive to the public, ensuring maximum uptake and efficacy in preventing the development of obesity or, as interventions, reducing obesity. Many are happening in both the health service and in the commercial sector. This is all good but there is a need to ensure that initiatives are effective, particularly if health service monies are to be invested.

Sometimes an initiative might appear likely to produce a successful outcome but on independent assessment this might not be the case.

To tackle obesity, a range of weight-loss programmes, within national healthcare systems or the private sector, have been established in response to, and to address, the growing obesity crisis. In the UK, in an attempt to improve outcomes and value for money, any scheme or programme funded from public money must fulfil a number of criteria outlined by the National Institute for Health and Clinical Excellence (NICE).[8]

There is considerable variability in the management of overweight and obese people within the NHS. In 2001, the National Audit Office report[9] identified that no central guidance on obesity management existed. Few health authorities (only 28%) had taken action to address obesity as a health problem for local populations. Certainly there was evidence that primary care played an important role in the management of obesity but general practitioners and practice nurses used a wide range of methods to manage overweight and obese patients and many were uncertain as to which interventions were most effective. Primary care was found to be willing to address the problem[10] yet the provision of services remained limited and inconsistent. Despite 55% of primary care organisations believing that prevention and treatment of obesity was a priority, only 31% had established a weight management clinic. The NAO report[9] found that primary care organisations (PCOs) had developed a number of innovative approaches to the management of obesity, including partnerships with local authority and commercial weight-loss organisations, but that there was considerable regional variation in service provision.

It should be remembered that a PCO could claim involvement in obesity-related interest despite only minimal activity in the field; the extent of their involvement was not assessed. As a result it is not surprising that most PCOs which did provide support and services for overweight and obese patients failed to monitor the effectiveness of these interventions. Only 19% monitored outcomes for surgery, 39% drug treatment, 45% weight loss and 15% for other interventions including dietetic and nutrition, physical activity programmes and exercise on prescription. Moreover, 91% offered exercise on prescription and 59% advice on 'healthy shopping'. Yet it is accepted that general practitioners, practice nurses and community pharmacists have little if any training in the delivery of service for this patient group.[11] There is a need to ensure the quality of the service provided to patients within the NHS; all services need to be fully scrutinised.

Obesity services

There are some encouraging developments in service delivery for obese and overweight patient groups and many examples of good practice exist. As healthcare professionals we need to stop re-inventing the wheel and adopt locally effective service for our patients or client groups, some clear service specification that can be adopted nationally and disseminated, and which will ensure that all patients, no matter where they live, will have access to services that will address their needs. And there is no reason why these services should be restricted to primary healthcare professionals. The private sector, where their service is shown to be effective, could be considered as a partner in addressing the problem.

Indeed the National Audit Office[9] highlighted the need for joint working with different agencies to facilitate cross-government initiatives to prevent obesity at both national and local level and the need to consider the broader environment in terms of its potential to support behavioural change. This is essential since obesity, or rather its development, is not always a medical problem and therefore the solution goes beyond the clinical setting and extends into the wider community through work in schools, workplaces and neighbourhoods.[11]

Programmes or interventions exist to address the obese and support a reduction of body weight; we know normalisation is not often practical and from a health point of view is not even necessary; 5–10% weight loss brings significant benefit. These programmes address primary prevention, secondary prevention and chronic management of the obese patient. It will be impossible for one programme to address all the needs of this complex public health problem. Yet together these programmes, coupled with myriad initiatives across government and wider society, might become a long-term solution to the problem.

Website services

A range of excellent, good-quality websites that are easily accessed and that provide quality objective information and support for professionals and individuals can be a help in the battle against obesity. A selection of these sites are highlighted in box 7.1.

Private sector programmes

As the obesity epidemic increases and becomes a greater threat to public health, there is renewed interest in using the weight management services on offer in the private sector to support the health service. To do this will require evidence that these services work. To date there is very little good-quality research into these programmes but reasonable evidence exists for meal replacement therapies, and diets such as Slimming World, Weight Watchers and the Rosemary Conley programme and very-low-energy diets such as Lighterlife. However, other products offered by the commercial

Box 7.1 Websites providing information on managing obesity

MEND
http://www.mendprogramme.org
A community-based, family-orientated childhood obesity programme emanating from Great Ormond Street

Leeds Metropolitan University/Carnegie Weight Management
http://carnegieweightmanagement.com/
Community-based weight-loss club programmes available through-out Britain.

National Obesity Forum
http://nationalobesityforum.org.uk/content/view/23/36/
Charity dedicated to raising awareness of obesity in the context of chronic disease, and improving its management in clinical care. It is currently setting up regional groups in the nine SHA regions of the UK, to improve obesity management and to facilitate PCTs in setting up appropriate obesity services.

International Diabetes Federation
http://www.idf.org/webdata/docs/IDF_Meta_def_final.pdf

British Heart Foundation
http://www.bhf.org.uk/

Diabetes UK
http://www.diabetes.org.uk/

Department of Health
http://www.dh.gov.uk/en/index.htm

British Nutrition Foundation
http://www.nutrition.org.uk/home.asp?siteId=43&sectionId=s

It's what you gain
http://www.itswhatyougain.co.uk/
Sponsored website that provides a range of resources, including weight management, risk prevention strategies and current treatment.

sector may be tainted by the past enthusiasm of their marketing departments which, rather than using results from properly designed clinical trials, often opted for personal testimonials from satisfied customers. Furthermore the science of such interventions, although previously flawed, is now validated by the Committee on the Medical Aspects of Food Policy and NICE and provides an extra means by which overweight and obese individuals can seek help. Increasingly dissatisfied customers are using the internet to make their disappointment with such programmes known, and for this reason, these organisations are becoming more appreciative of the need for quality and a sound evidence base.

Diet trials

Diet Trials, a high-profile study undertaken in the UK, documented in a BBC series, compared the effectiveness of four commercial weight-loss diets in a group of adults. The trial period was 6 months, assessing around 300 over-weight or obese subjects who were randomly assigned to one of the diets or a control.[12] It was therefore a randomised, unblinded, controlled trial and took place in a community-based sample of otherwise healthy adults.

The diets assessed were:

- Dr Atkins' New Diet Revolution
- Slim-Fast
- Weight Watchers Pure Points programme
- Rosemary Conley's Eat Yourself Slim diet

All diets resulted in significant loss of body fat and weight over 6 months. This well-designed study found that groups did not differ significantly at the end of the study period but loss of body fat and weight was greater in all groups compared with the control group. Average weight loss was 5.9 kg and average fat loss was 4.4 kg over 6 months. The Atkins diet resulted in significantly higher weight loss during the first 4 weeks but by the end was no more effective than the other diets.

The conclusion was that clinically useful weight loss and fat loss can be achieved in adults who are motivated to follow commercial diets for a substantial period. Given the limited resources for weight management in the NHS, healthcare practitioners should discuss with their patients programmes known to be effective.

Researchers identified few significant differences in cardiac risk factors between the diets groups and the control group. Initially, the fall in systolic pressure in the Atkins group was significantly greater than in the Slim-Fast group but not the other groups, probably because of the relatively greater initial weight loss in the Atkins group. Glucose concentrations fell slightly over time; only in the Weight Watchers group was fasting glucose significantly lower than in the control group. In the first two months, a significant but small drop in total cholesterol was seen in all diet groups except for the Atkins group. By 6 months, cholesterol had fallen significantly compared with the control group only in the Weight Watchers group (by 0.55 mmol/l).

A secondary analysis of data from participants who completed the trial shows the range of weight lost by these highly motivated participants, who probably adhered most strongly to the randomly allocated diets; some participants lost more than 25 kg yet others gained weight.

After 6 months all diets resulted in a clinically useful mean reduction in percentage body weight:

- Rosemary Conley diet: 9.9%
- Weight Watchers: 9.0%
- Atkins: 8.9%
- Slim-Fast: 6.8%.

The proportion of participants who completed the trial and lost at least 10% of their body weight at 6 months was 46% for the Rosemary Conley group, 45% for the Atkins group, 36% for the Weight Watchers group, and 21% for the Slim-Fast group. These losses were achieved despite the random allocation of diets.

The range of absolute weight loss in participants who completed the study was wide. Compliance was variable and correlated with successful outcome. Compliance with each diet varied greatly and since some of the participants took part in the television documentary it is not clear what effect this publicity had on compliance.

Primary care based programmes

Rotherham obesity strategy and Rotherham Institute for Obesity

The Rotherham obesity strategy for the management of adult obesity involves three tiers of intervention. The initial level of intervention is a time-limited, 12-week programme of diet, nutrition, lifestyle and exercise advice provided by trained staff under the supervision and management of the local Rotherham dietetics department. Those patients who do not lose sufficient weight in this initial intervention, or who need more specialist intervention because they are considered to be more at risk of cardiometabolic conse-quences associated with obesity, are referred into the middle tier of inter-vention. This is provided by the Rotherham Institute for Obesity (RIO) under the clinical management of Dr Matt Capehorn. Those adults considered to have other health problems that may be complicated by their obesity or that are influencing the effectiveness of their weight management programme, are referred to the third tier of intervention, which involves secondary care (hospital) input with the relevant speciality. This secondary care input may in some cases include bariatric surgery for those patients considered to be most at risk and who meet local as well as national criteria.

The Rotherham childhood obesity model also follows a tiered approach. The initial level of intervention is provided by existing local resources pro-vided by general practitioners, dieticians, health visitors, school nurses etc.

Those children considered to be too overweight for their given age, as defined by established child growth charts, are referred into a local programme of 'Carnegie Clubs' provided by locally trained staff under the guidance and expertise of the Carnegie Weight Management programme based at the Leeds Metropolitan University. Those children considered to be unsuccessful at this level of intervention are also referred to the RIO to receive more specialist weight management input and advice as part of a family-based approach. A certain number of those children considered to be most at risk each year are referred on to attend the 'Carnegie Camps', or residential weight management programmes provided by Carnegie Weight Management.

The RIO is a specialist centre for the management of obesity. It forms the basis of the middle tier of intervention for adults and children with weight management problems, as part of the overall Rotherham obesity strategy. It has a multidisciplinary team approach to managing weight problems by providing specialists in all aspects of the current thinking in weight management. This includes dedicated obesity specialist nurses, healthcare assistants, dieticians, psychologist and counsellors, health activity specialist, a general practitioner with a specialist interest in obesity, and access to regular sessions with a bariatric surgeon and other secondary care specialists.

It is intended that most patients who require the services provided by RIO will be those who have received the initial tier of weight management intervention offered locally but considered unsuccessful in their level of weight loss. Patients can also be referred directly to RIO via local general practitioners, or medical practitioners at the local hospital, if they meet specific criteria that deem them to be particularly at risk of the cardio-metabolic consequences of obesity, or need any of the more specialist intervention offered by RIO. It is hoped that in the future, further care pathways can be developed to allow referrals for patients who may have accessed, yet been unsuccessful in, other accredited weight management programmes that may be offered locally by pharmacists or in the private sector.

When patient referrals are initially received, they are triaged to assess which, if not all, of the services offered by RIO are required, and appointments made as appropriate. All patients are initially assessed in a dedicated weighing and measuring room and all parameters including blood pressure, weight, height, body mass index (BMI), and fat composition using bio-impedance scales are taken. Regularly calibrated weigh-bridge scales are used in order to provide consistency of measurements for weights of morbidly obese levels, and for patients with limited mobility. If no recent blood tests have been performed, these are taken on-site, to exclude previously undiagnosed metabolic conditions or associated risk factors.

All patients receive further basic dietary and nutritional advice as well as lifestyle and exercise education throughout the length of time they are in the service. This may include further explanation of the specific roles of calories, portion sizes and nights off the diet, or education on basic cooking skills in order to complement nutritional advice given (provided in on-site kitchen facilities). There are opportunities to discuss other aspects of their lives with health trainers, counsellors proficient in techniques such as cognitive behavioural therapy or neurolinguistic programming, or a psychologist. Appointments with an activity specialist help tailor specific exercise programmes suitable for the individual (provided in on-site gym facilities). Patients who are to be considered for pharmacotherapy are assessed by the general practitioner with a specialist interest in obesity for a review of their co-existing medical conditions and medications. When appropriate, medications are provided on normal FP10 NHS prescriptions which are charged to the drug budget of the patient's own general practitioner. Consultations are performed on a one-to-one basis in dedicated consulting rooms. Further facilities within the institute include a dedicated meeting room, which allows group work or educational meetings for patients or healthcare professionals. This room provides a resource library with computer terminals, and obesity-related books, journals and other educational tools. It is hoped that in the future the service will work with other centres to form part of further research into the management of obesity.

Patients going through the RIO service are considered a success if they meet certain criteria depending on the individual. For example, for most patients this may be considered to be 3–5% weight loss at 3 months, maintained at 6 months. For other patients it may be more; however, in the case of certain children, weight maintenance alone may be an achievable goal. A further role for RIO could be in the preoperative and postoperative care for patients requiring referral for bariatric surgery. In this way a fluid and integrated service in both directions through the tiers of the overall obesity strategy can be maintained. It is hoped that patient data will be recorded on a population database within RIO, irrespective of what tier of service a patient happens to be in at any given time. Long term data can thus be obtained for all patients accessing the Rotherham obesity service, at any level of intervention. Results from the service will be regularly audited and the overall Rotherham obesity strategy is subject to a regular monitoring process by service providers and members of NHS Rotherham. The Rotherham obesity strategy may be accessed by all of the 250 000 population of Rotherham. Patients can now finally have the opportunity to be prescribed a trip to RIO!

Counterweight programme

Counterweight is an evaluated, evidence-based primary care weight-management programme currently provided throughout Scotland, and in an increasing number of English and Welsh primary care trusts (PCTs). It is a nurse-led programme that equips general practitioners and practice nurses to provide evidence-based approaches to weight management. It employs a structured approach to care and an interactive model of communication designed to empower patients. Between 2000 and 2005 the programme was piloted in 80 UK general practices and is currently being rolled out.

Counterweight is commissioned through PCTs in England (usually in blocks of 10 practices) whereas in Scotland the programme is funded centrally by the government and is available mainly through general practitioner practices, in all health boards across the country. Counterweight is designed to incorporate a weight management service into existing healthcare services. The objective of the programme is simple and is primarily to achieve and maintain a medically valuable weight loss of between 5% and 10% for as many people as possible. It is a flexible and sustainable model and can be adapted to deliver tailored programmes to individuals, groups or families, depending on need and the level of resources available. Although evaluated in a primary care (general practitioner practice setting) it can be adapted for use in other settings. In Scotland there is some interest in providing the service through community pharmacy.

Within the Counterweight model that patients can opt to undertake are a goal-setting approach, a structured, prescribed eating plan or a group programme, all based on a daily energy deficit of 500–600 kcal. The use of a number of behavioural strategies is a core component of the Counterweight model, which also incorporates advice on increasing physical activity. The intervention programme is a structured pathway for management of obesity in primary care, consisting of screening and evidence-based treatment guidelines.

The programme incorporates evidence-based care pathways and strategies to empower clinicians and patients. The model is based on weight management advisers (dieticians specialising in obesity management) working across PCTs, training and supporting practice staff to put the Counterweight programme into practice. It is anticipated that each trained practice could treat an average of 50 patients each year. Each patient is recommended to have nine appointments of 10–30 minutes duration in the first year.

Lifestyle intervention is recommended as a first-line approach to weight management, delivered individually or in groups; second line interventions may include the use of anti-obesity medications, referral to a dietitian, psychologist and/or a secondary care services. Weight maintenance is encouraged, either following weight loss or as the first option with particular groups of patients.

Counterweight is tailored to suit local priorities, services and available personnel and it is designed to integrate into a wider obesity management strategy involving key stakeholders from primary and secondary care. Within primary care the whole team including general practitioners, nurses, surgery-assistants, dieticians, practice managers and receptionists should be engaged in decisions regarding implementation of the programme. Locally employed 'buddy' dieticians are involved in order to take over responsibility for Counterweight once the model has been implemented. Training an additional NHS dietitian could provide support for five extra practices in the first 18 months and sustain the model in the following years.[13]

Evaluation

The service has been assessed. Mean weight change at 12 months was a 3.0 kg weight reduction in all patients (n = 684, p < 0.001) and a 4.3 kg weight reduction in high attenders (n = 422, p < 0.001). At 24 months, weight change was 2.4 kg reduction in all patients (n = 391, p < 0.001) and 3.3 kg reduction in high attenders (n = 225, p < 0.001). Thirty per cent of all patients enrolled and were followed up in the programme, and almost 40% of high attenders maintained 5% loss or more at 12 months (figure 7.1).

There is also compelling evidence that weight loss is highly beneficial in reducing the risk of serious chronic disease and the data reported by the Counterweight programme provides the 'missing link', proving that the induction and maintenance of weight loss is possible across a population 'in the wild' in primary care, and is both clinically effective and cost effective.[14-16] The provision of Counterweight in clinical care certainly costs less than ignoring weight management altogether. The evaluation of the cost effectiveness of the Counterweight programme used an economic model originally developed to provide input to the UK national guidance on

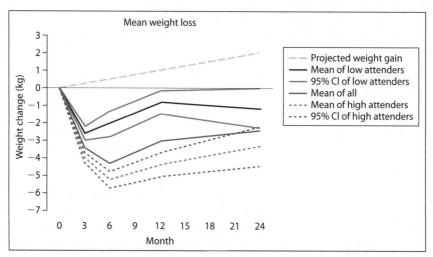

Figure 7.1 Mean weight loss for all patients, high and low attenders.

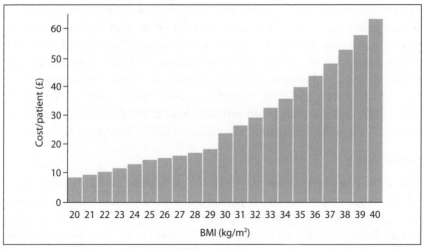

Figure 7.2 Impact of BMI on prescribing costs of 'top 10' drugs (males).

obesity. It was developed by NICE and the £57 cost per QALY (quality-adjusted life year) for Counterweight proves it to be excellent value for money. In comparison the cost per QALY for smoking cessation is £700 and the accepted benchmark for cost effectiveness in the UK is £20 000–30 000 per QALY.

Obesity is associated with increasing prescribing costs across all categories of the formulary, and deliberate loss of weight is linked to reduced costs of pharmaceutical agents (figure 7.2).

Effect of Counterweight intervention on prescribing costs

By applying the mean change in BMI observed in the pilot phase of Counterweight to the costs of prescribing at varying BMI levels, expected savings can be estimated. These savings were 6.3% of prescribing costs for all patients and 8.4% of prescribing costs for patients whose attendance with the programme was optimal. Attributable prescribing costs of obesity were calculated by applying cost at BMI >30 kg/m^2 minus cost at normal weight, multiplying up by the population of the UK and showing that as a proportion of total prescribing costs:

- 16% of the total prescribing costs can be attributable to obesity
- 26% of the total prescribing costs can be attributable to overweight and obesity.

After applying the percentage savings estimated from weight loss observed with the Counterweight programme, it can be concluded that in Year 1 alone, 10% of the cost of the programme can be offset through prescribing savings (this figure increasing to 25% when programme attendance and follow up is optimal).

Longer term cost-effectiveness

Applying the NICE model to evaluate the long-term impact demonstrates that providing primary care obesity management is cheaper and more effective than providing no weight management intervention:

- Prescribing costs increase with increasing BMI.
- Weight change outcomes observed in the Counterweight programme will bring associated cost savings.
- One-quarter of all prescribing costs can be attributed to overweight and obesity.
- Longer term analysis shows that providing Counterweight is cheaper and more effective than doing nothing.

MEND programme

The MEND (Mind, Exercise, Nutrition, Do it!) is a programme focused on families with children aged 7–13 years whose weight is above the healthy range for their age and height. The programme was developed at the Great Ormond Street Hospital for Children and the University College London, Institute of Child Health. The programme runs twice a week after school in 2-hour sessions over 10 weeks, that is, 20 sessions in all. Each session comprises an hour of physical activity and a 1-hour interactive session on nutritional topics and activity. Currently over 300 programmes are provided weekly across the UK through a partnership approach with private, public and not-for-profit organisations.

The objective of the programme is to help children and families manage their weight better and to lead healthier lives. Those families who engage with the MEND programme are taught the basics of good nutrition and eating a balanced diet as well as learning how to be more active. The programme also addresses motivation and provides some motivational techniques. This ensures that lifestyles changes are supported and become normalised within day-to-day behaviour. In particular, attitudes to food and exercise are addressed so that changes are sustained in the long-term. MEND is not a diet programme and expressly does not encourage rapid weight loss, focusing instead on practical issues, fun and learning designed to deliver sustainable improvement in family diet, fitness and overall health.

Evaluation

Over 5000 overweight and obese children and their parents have now attended the MEND programme, which makes it the UK's largest family and community-based intervention for childhood obesity. The MEND programme has an evidence base that shows that it helps children lose weight, particularly body fat, increases their physical activity levels and self-esteem and reduces their sedentary behaviours such as the time they spend watching television or playing computer games. The MEND programme is effective in achieving statistically significant and sustained improvements in key health outcomes at 12 months such as BMI, waist circumference, increased participation in and uptake of physical activity and reduced sedentary behaviour as well as sustainable improvements in self-esteem.[17]

Healthy Weight Challenge

There are a number of effective pharmacy-based weight management services documented internationally.[18–20]

A small, community pharmacy-based pilot – the Healthy Weight Challenge – was set up in 2002 in partnership with a local community group, the Falls Women's Centre in Belfast, Northern Ireland. The initiative is funded by the Building the Community Pharmacy Partnership, a government-funded body that supported community development.

The community pharmacy's contribution to the programme was:

- to promote healthy eating and exercise generally to the local community
- to facilitate those who are overweight or obese to identify and then achieve their healthy weight.

The centre provided 'evening classes' (a series of meetings addressing different aspects of obesity and how to avoid it). In addition, the centre provide trained counsellors to assist individuals who have specific personal or social problems that might be contributing to excessive energy intake.

The pilot project was completed in January 2004 and provided some encouraging results and the basis on which a more clearly defined community pharmacy-based service might be developed.

The Healthy Weight Challenge was advertised by leaflet and a newspaper advertisement, and members of the public were asked to enrol. Those wishing to join were offered advice on a healthy diet and taking more exercise. Their blood pressure, blood glucose and serum cholesterol was measured. Those with a BMI of over 30 kg/m^2 were offered one-to-one support to achieve a target weight and those who had major life-issues were offered counselling and support from the counsellors working for the women's centre.

The results were encouraging. Of the 168 people enrolled, 35 were invited to take part in the programme all of whom had a BMI of 35 kg/m^2 or more. The programme involved weekly interventions: advice on diet, nutrition and exercise, and target setting for weight and monitoring. At 6 months 13% had lost 8–12 kg, 8% had lost more than 12 kg and 11% had either stayed the same or gained some weight. No drug therapy was used in the programme.[21]

Coventry pharmacy obesity service

Based on the Healthy Weight Challenge pilot, the Coventry Pharmacy Obesity Service was designed to develop and further pilot the benefits of a pharmacy-based obesity service within a single primary care organisation (Coventry Primary Care Trust) and to access the impact of this service with a view of using it as an enhanced service specification within the new pharmacy contract for England.

Development

A panel of experts was convened to develop the structure and specifications for the pharmacy-based obesity service and initially it used the template from the Health Weight Challenge[21] as the basis of the service specification, with modifications applied taking account of local clinical guidelines.

The aim was to provide an obesity management service for patients over the age of 18 years, with a BMI of between 30 and 38 kg/m^2, with at least *one* diagnosed or established risk factor. The risk factors include:

- hypertension
- type 2 diabetes
- hyperlipidaemia
- increased waist circumference – greater than 102 cm for males and more than 88 cm for women. (For Asian men the measurement should be below 90 cm and for Asian women below 80 cm.)

Enrolment of pharmacies

Pharmacies were enrolled by PCT selection following a letter to all contractors within the PCT. A minimum requirement was a commitment to the programme, completion of the training and an agreement to enrol a defined number of overweight or obese patients who would be monitored over 12 months.

Training

Two training events were organised to support pharmacists delivering the service. Training covered the main areas of competence required by the average practising pharmacist: epidemiology of obesity, obesity and disease risk, change management (mainly motivational interviewing technique), nutrition, exercise, using clinical testing equipment and recording data.

Methodology

Accredited pharmacists enrolled patients with the support of a media campaign and poster leaflet display by the PCT. They also actively enrolled patients in the pharmacy when dealing with them in a professional capacity. For example, a patient with type 2 diabetes who visited the pharmacy to collect medication and who was clearly overweight would be asked 'How are you getting on managing your weight?' The pharmacist was trained to respond appropriately based on the response:

- If the patient was dismissive, the pharmacist backed off.
- If the patient was interested, a brief intervention was initiated using motivational interviewing.
- If the patient was keen to do something, she was offered the weight management programme.

Enhanced service

The one-to-one service used a proforma template to record data on each enrolled patient and included: BMI, waist circumference, blood glucose, total cholesterol and blood pressure. Referrals were made to the patient's general practitioner where any results were outside normal values, as determined by local guidelines.

A food diary was discussed with the client to identify areas of excess energy intake and activity, and exercise was discussed. As a minimum, government guidelines on nutrition and exercise were given within advice and was supported by written leaflets.

A target weight was set for the patient. This normally corresponded to a 5–10% reduction in weight over a minimum period of 6 months. A reduction in energy intake equivalent to 600 kcal daily was agreed, along with an exercise programme (a minimum of 30 minutes of moderate exercise on 5 days in the week).

Each patient enrolled was followed up initially every 2 weeks for 1 month, then monthly up to 6 months and then bi-monthly up to 12 months. At each subsequent meeting, the nutrition and exercise information was reinforced, measurements were repeated and progress monitored.

Evaluation

The primary outcome for this service was a minimum of 5% reduction in BMI and waist circumference. The pilot was completely based on a one-to-one intervention based on behavioural change and did not involve the use of weight reduction medicines – indeed, these were a contraindication for enrolment. There was, as with any behaviour intervention service, a fall off in follow up as the project proceeded, with only approximately 30% of participants providing data at 12 months. The reason for this failure to follow up was not clearly explained but often other priorities replace attendance, as individuals may assess that they no longer need help and are able to help themselves. At 6 months, 112 patients had been enrolled into the service and 72 patients had completed four follow ups and had lost on average 0.618 of their BMI and an average 3.37 cm of waist circumference.

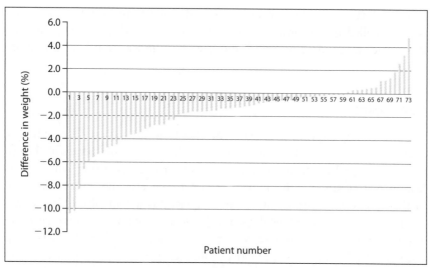

Figure 7.3 Percentage difference in weight of patients.

The average BMI at recruitment was $34.4\,kg/m^2$. Of the 112 patients recruited, 80% (n = 59) have had a reduction in weight from recruitment until follow up and 20% (n = 15) have had a slight increase in BMI since recruitment (figure 7.3). Of the patients who have shown a reduction in weight, 14% (n = 8) lost 5% or more of their recruitment weight, which is in line with service objectives.

There were 38 general practitioner referrals, for 53 monitoring parameters that were out of range. One referral was made to the Senior Clinical Exercise Physiologist. A breakdown is shown in figure 7.4.

Twenty-six per cent of participants had achieved a weight loss of 5% or more at 12 months. The average change in weight was a loss of 3.7 kg, (n = 34). Similarly, the mean change in BMI at 12 months was a reduction of $1.3\,kg/m^2$ (n = 34). The mean change in waist circumference at 12 months was an average reduction of 6.69 cm (n = 34).[20]

This pharmacy-based obesity management service has proven that community pharmacies are well placed to provide a weight management

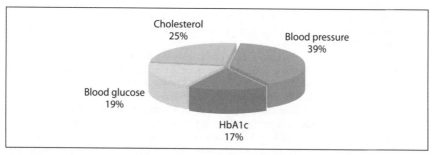

Figure 7.4 Number of referrals made by pharmacists to general practitioners.

service effectively, and to achieve statistically significant results. The service is being rolled out to other PCTs across England and there are plans that this service might become an enhanced service, under the title of a vascular service.

Conclusion

To address the growing prevalence of obesity and to assist those who are overweight and obese, there is a need for a range of easily accessible health promotion, health education and intervention initiatives that will address healthy eating and taking more exercise to be effective in avoiding the further development of obesity. At its simplest this will involve media advertising, posters, window displays and leaflets. It might also involve more innovative use of weighting scales, the calculation of BMI and waist-to-hip ratio calculation in clinical practice. There clearly is a role for the private sector but there will be a need to ensure that where public money is used, proper evaluation is undertaken.

References

1. Diabetes Prevention Programme Research Group. Reduction in the incidence of type 2 diabetes with lifestyle intervention or metformin. *New Engl J Med* 2002; 346: 393–403.
2. Tuomilehto J *et al.* Prevention of type 2 diabetes mellitus by changes in lifestyle among subjects with impaired glucose tolerance. *New Engl J Med* 2001; 344: 1343–1349.
3. Wei M *et al.* Waist circumference as the best predictor of (NIDDM) compared to BMI, waist/hip ratio and other anthropometric measurements in Mexican Americans: A 7-year prospective study. *Obes Res* 1997; 5: 16–23.
4. National Heart, Lung and Blood Institute. *The Practical Guide. Identification, evaluation and treatment of overweight and obesity in adults.* Bethesda, MD: National Institutes of Health, 1998.
5. Broom J *et al.* Systematic review of the long term outcomes of the treatments for obesity and implication for health improvement and the economic consequences for the National Health Service. *Health Technology Assessment* 2004, vol. 8, no. 21.
6. King M *et al.* Foresight Project Report. *Tackling Obesities: future choices.* London: Government Office For Science, 2007.
7. Templeton S-K. Antiobesity drive to use shock tactic. *The Times Online* 9 Nov 2008. http://www.timesonline.co.uk/tol/life_and_style/health/article5114359.ece (accessed 10 Jul 2009).
8. National Institute for Health and Clinical Excellence. Obesity: the prevention, identification, assessment and management of overweight and obesity in adults and children. *Clinical Guidance* 2006; 43.
9. National Audit Office. *Tackling Obesity in England.* London: NAO, 2001.
10. Dr Foster Report. Primary care management of adult obesity in the UK, 2005. http://www.drfosterintelligence.co.uk (accessed 22 Nov 2008).
11. Garrow D, Summerbell H. Penalties of shifting weight. *BMJ* 1995; 311: 1653–1654.
12. Truby H *et al.* Randomised controlled trial of four commercial weight loss programmes in the UK: initial findings from the BBC "diet trials" *BMJ* 2006; 332: 1309–1314.
13. National Institute for Health and Clinical Excellence. *Obesity: guidance on the prevention, identification, assessment and management of overweight and obesity in adults and*

children. NICE Clinical Guideline No. 43. London: NICE, 2006. http://www.nice.org.uk/ CG043 (accessed 10 Jul 2008).

14. Counterweight Project Team. A new evidence-based model for weight management in primary care: the Counterweight Programme. *J Hum Nutr Diet* 2004; 17: 191–208.

15. Counterweight Project Team. Evaluation of the Counterweight Programme for obesity management in primary care: a starting point for continuous improvement. *Br J Gen Pract* 2008; 548–554.

16. Counterweight Project Team. An economic evaluation of the Counterweight Programme in the United Kingdom. *Circulation* 2007; 116: II-822.

17. Sacher P M *et al*. The MEND RCT. Effectiveness on health outcomes in obese children. *Int J Obes* 2007; 31: S1.

18. Ahrens R *et al*. The role of pharmacy in obesity management. *J Am Pharm Assoc* 2003; 43: 583–589.

19. Malone M *et al*. Obesity management: a role for pharmacy. *Ann Pharmacother* 2003; 37: 1598–1602.

20. Glare J. Obesity services development in pharmacy. *JAMA* 2008; 299: 1139–1148.

21. Shah M. *et al*. Obesity management in primary care; The Coventry Project. A report to the Chief Pharmacist. Chessington: Unichem Ltd, 2008.

8

Behavioural interventions

Chapter 7 considered the spectrum of services offered that address the obesity problem. At the core of all of these services is behavioural modification. This chapter discusses behavioural modification techniques that are effective when a primary care practitioner is working one-to-one with a patient or client or working in a group context.

Our behaviours are the outcome of our decisions on the choices available to us, and ultimately result from taking one course of action as opposed to another. Our decisions are arrived at mainly through a combination of conscious and subconscious processes that, in a crude way, are a cost-benefit analysis about engaging, or not, in a given activity. This may seem an exaggeration or oversophistication of what is really a simplistic process as most of our behaviours appear to be reflective. Yet much of this decision-making process is determined or preconditioned by past experiences, the opinions of significant others (peers) and the options on offer in our environment. Behaviours are also highly influenced by our personal beliefs and values, although they may also seem reflective.

Role in weight management

Behavioural therapy for obesity was first developed in the 1950s, at the same time that Dr Albert Stunkard in America started to realise that patients with binge eater disorder and night eating syndrome had no chance of responding to the mere suggestion of 'going on a diet', but that intensive counselling and psychological input was required. The prevailing theory at the time was that the root cause of obesity was an 'obese eating style'.[1] Behavioural therapy would, so the theory went, ensure a return to normal body weight by eliminating abnormal eating behaviours, and normal weight would be sustained permanently.

Although this initial expectation has been proved to be a little optimistic, behavioural techniques have improved, and with the advent of cognitive behavioural therapy (CBT) in the 1970s, to identify and manage negative thoughts, a role for CBT has emerged in long-term obesity management. In addition, motivational interviewing technique (MIT) was developed in the

1990s as a patient-centred, directional counselling technique and is proving successful in many areas of obesity management.

Behavioural therapy is one of the three traditional facets of obesity management, the others being diet and physical activity but, unlike diet and exercise, behavioural therapy is poorly understood by most healthcare professionals, who often do not develop the necessary skills to apply it in practice. It is true that many behavioural psychologists and therapists have tended to overcomplicate the art but that should not be used as a reason to ignore behavioural therapy as an effective tool in obesity management.

If a person arrives home late from a stressful day at work and heads straight to the fridge for half a pound of cheese, then basic dietary advice would be 'Stop doing that, it's very bad for you' but behavioural therapy might suggest ways how not to eat the cheese. The answer might be surprisingly easy advice: 'Don't buy cheese'; or more complex: 'Avoid the stressful situation that triggered the desire for the cheese', which may mean getting a new job, or taking a relaxing walk home instead of travelling by overcrowded public transport. Other suggestions might include not putting the cheese at the front of the fridge where it is seen as soon as the door is opened to get milk for a cup of tea; or have readily accessible healthy snacks, such as fruit, to hand instead. Alternatively there may be other means of relaxation, such as going for a run or having a bath. Behavioural therapy covers the range of techniques and strategies used to bring about changes in lifestyle and should always be used in the context of traditional dietary and physical activity advice in order to maximize the overall benefits.

In the context of obesity, behaviours, such as our eating habits and engagement, or not, with physical activity, are clearly of primacy. In general those who are obese or are becoming obese, are so mainly as a result of their dietary and activity behaviours. As a result, successfully addressing an individual's obesity, and as a consequence reducing their risk of disease, necessitates modification of current behaviours. Although this sounds simple enough, in terms of effecting behaviour change, humans prove particularly resistant.

Behaviour choices

Humans are genetically 'hardwired' to seek comfort and avoid pain.[1] In this way a simplistic model of human behaviour might suppose that when someone considers engaging in, or avoiding, a behaviour, the final decision (usually 'avoid') will be based on a complex assessment of the costs and benefits to the individual.

Perception of risk

For obesity, unhealthy behaviours might include: eating too many calories; choosing foods poor in nutritional value; spending hours seated in front of the television; taking the lift rather than walking up stairs and so on. The short-term benefits of these behaviours to the individual are obvious. Failure to adopt healthier behaviours that will normalise body weight such as eating fewer calories, choosing more nutritious foods and taking more exercise might reflect ignorance of the facts – but even when facts are provided, and understood, there still may be a failure to adapt, perhaps because the long-term cost of the behaviour is given insufficient priority.

Chapter 7 discusses the use of government public health campaigns to support behavioural change – Edwina Currie, then health minister, all but destroyed the UK's egg industry by announcing, unintentionally, that the national egg-laying flock was infected with *Salmonella*. The abrupt halt in egg consumption was in sharp contrast to a high-profile, government-sponsored public health campaign aimed at encouraging people to eat at most two eggs per week because of the increased risk of heart disease, which failed dismally to reduce consumption. The risk of acute diarrhoea today was perceived as unacceptable, whereas the risk of a heart attack in 20 years' time somehow seemed tolerable. Individuals are highly motivated to change behaviour when presented with an acute potential risk yet relatively uncon-cerned about a future risk.

Default options

The environment in which we live greatly dictates the range of options avail-able to us and in this way has a considerable effect on our behaviours. Where human beings are programmed by our evolution to seek out pleasure and avoid pain, we are also programmed to save energy and making a decision requires energy. We are lazy when it comes to decision making; we are more likely to take the 'default option', i.e. the option that least requires a decision to be made particularly if that decision refers to some long-term benefit. A study of workers and their participation in company pension schemes – a decision that will only have long-term benefits to the individual – gives some insight to this fact. Where workers in a company had to opt into a company pension scheme only 25% did so whereas where the workers were required to opt out of the company pension scheme some 79% remained in the scheme and were happy with monthly payments.[2] This is an important insight as it highlights the fact that individuals are more likely to make a behaviour choice because that choice is the easiest one to make; it requires least effort. Where a moving escalator is provided alongside a staircase it is not unusual to find that most people choose to take the escalator rather than the stairs; the escalator becomes the default option as it is easier, it requires least effort.

Fast-food outlets provide easy access to high-energy foods and they are highly visible on the high street of every town and city and at transport stations between cities. Where a healthy option is unavailable, or is not as palatable, it is not surprising that people will choose a default option, that is, to eat in a fast-food establishment. In addition, road policy, particularly in the US, even allows shoppers to avoid getting out of their cars at retail outlets and, if they do not have to, the short-term benefits – conserving energy – will far outweigh the long-term risk of putting on weight. In our modern, highly obesogenic environments, we have implemented options to make life easier: television remote controls, automatic doors, emails, mobile phones, even central heating. The default option is the option that requires the least energy and the least decision to be made. Today we expend less energy and we get easier access to food than all previous generations.

Changing behaviour

Much of the work on behaviour, and behavioural change, and most of the theoretical models that have been proposed from this work, has been undertaken by psychologists and over the years an impressive, and sometimes confusing, list of theories and models has emerged. These have been critically assessed by Robert West, a clinical psychologist, and a detailed consideration of the myriad theories is beyond the scope of this chapter.[3]

Context

Supporting and facilitating behavioural change can be difficult and frustrating for healthcare professionals. People often seem to know and appreciate the dangers of continuing with certain behaviours, such as not taking enough exercise or eating too many calories, yet seem incapable of changing their lifestyles to reduce their health risk. In theory, change for individuals involves passing through a series of stages, the speed of passage differing between individuals; some pass through the stages so fast as to suggest the process is 'spontaneous', others take a considerable time and at some stages appear to get 'stuck'. What is known from research is that opportunistic brief advice and/or brief interventions by healthcare professionals are as effective in bringing about significant behaviour change as more prolonged counselling programmes.[4] In this way it is essential that all healthcare professionals, including pharmacists and their support staff, use every opportunity of professional contact to support and facilitate beneficial behavioural change and in this way reduce disease risk from obesity.

Supporting behavioural change to reduce disease risk is a central plank in the UK. Public health policy and has spawned major initiatives such as 'health action zones' and other community plans such as the introduction of health trainers as well as a greater requirement for healthcare professionals to work actively with individuals and communities. These are focused on the adoption of healthier behaviours through change.

Government White Papers such as *Choosing Health* (2004)[5] and *Our Health, Our Care, Our Say* (2006)[6] commit to this policy and are driving local initiatives to support and to facilitate behavioural change as a means of improving public health.

In the UK, community pharmacy is already supporting these initiatives within a national strategy outlined in *Choosing Health through Pharmacy: a programme for pharmaceutical public health 2005–2015*[7] emphasising the role for community pharmacy. This will support the distribution of guidance and support material and of course will be underpinned by the new pharmacy contract.

Brief advice or brief intervention?

The Department of Health in the UK has, perhaps arbitrarily, defined brief advice and brief interventions to describe what approach healthcare professionals should take when opportunistically discussing health and lifestyle with an individual. Rather than being discrete activities, what government is attempting to do is to define a continuum that, according to the evidence base, is most likely to achieve a positive outcome.[4]

Brief advice is proactively and opportunistically raising and assessing a person's willingness to engage in further discussion about a healthy lifestyle issue. This may only take a few moments, certainly where the individual expresses an unwillingness to discuss the issue, or it might take up to 3 minutes, not normally longer. For example, a woman who is obviously overweight and perhaps obese may be in the pharmacy collecting her repeat prescription for metformin tablets. While advising her on the medicines, or perhaps performing a medicines-use review, the pharmacist might tactfully raise the issue of nutrition. For example, the pharmacist might say: 'Have you been advised by a nutritionist about healthy eating?'.

The response will indicate if the customer is willing to listen to the message. Where her response is dismissive, aggressive even, then it is best to back off immediately before resistance is created. If the woman expresses concern that the diet is designed to make her lose weight but it is not working then further discussion is possible.

Brief intervention is undertaken where someone responds positively to opportunistic proactive brief advice or specifically asks for help with a health-related issue. A brief intervention is targeted at supporting behavioural change and may involve offering a specialist service such as enrolment into a local smoking-cessation clinic or obesity programme. In this way signposting is one possible outcome of brief intervention. In practice, brief intervention normally involve 5–10 minutes with the client but can take up to 30 minutes. In the national smoking standard this is analogous to a level 2 intervention.

According to these definitions, brief advice is normally what the healthcare professional will do first. A negative response: 'You've got to die sometime!' will result at best in the offer of help in the future. Where the client is keen for more information, the interview moves onto a brief intervention if time is available or is stopped, with a request to return for a brief intervention when next visiting.

Promoting change

Human behaviours are embedded in individuals' values and beliefs. They strongly influence lifestyles and in turn contribute to disease risk. Change, by choosing healthier options and adopting healthier lifestyles, reduces risk to our health. This is self-evident. Stopping smoking reduces the risk of early death by some 25% and taking sufficient exercise and avoiding obesity will reduce our individual risk of developing type 2 diabetes mellitus by as much as 50%. So there exists a compelling evidence base that changing behaviours promotes good health.

But change is difficult to bring about and to sustain. To get people to stop their substance or alcohol abuse, reduce their calorie intake, increase their exercise, or to quit smoking, requires them to change and change is a complex internal process. The factors that create strongly held views and endorse beliefs and behaviours – 'MMR vaccine is not safe'; 'I just have a very sweet-tooth' – are more subtle and complex than they first appear.

Promoting change, and knowing how to support it and bring it about, is an important skill for pharmacists and other primary healthcare professionals and is fundamental to our professional responsibility to our patients. A smoker prescribed a proton pump inhibitor is less likely to achieve a cure for his gastro-oesophageal reflux disease while he continues to smoke. A woman with diabetes who fails to reduce her weight will have difficulty in controlling her diabetes, despite medication. The person showing poor concordance, who fails to take her or his medicine, runs the risk of their disease worsening significantly. 'If you keep on doing what you've always done, you'll keep on getting what you've always got.' (WL Bateman).

Just tell them!

Even where change brings clear health benefits, and people are informed accordingly, motivation to change can prove disappointing. Put simply, the very act of telling someone what to do often, itself, leads to failure. When this happens, pharmacists and other members of the pharmacy workforce can lose motivation and stop trying.

'They just don't listen so why should I waste my time?' How many times have you felt or said this?

To lose weight and to sustain weight loss, people must change and adopt a new lifestyle: eat fewer calories and introduce some form of daily exercise. Change is easy to describe but difficult to implement. Individuals will also show different responses to change.

Build a 'Big Why'

Why people change or do not change is a hugely complex area and theories abound.[3] The intention to change is dependent on three factors:

- attitude (I want to lose weight)
- subjective norm (What do the people whom I trust and care about think?)
- control (Can I do it?).

The philosopher Nietzsche's view that people will endure any 'how' when they are fully committed to the 'why' is an important insight in the context of attitude to change. In this way the role of the healthcare professional must be to foster, support then build a 'Big Why'. The more the individual sees what he or she wants in the future and the more they understand why they want it then 'the how', the means of achieving it, becomes much easier. This must be core to health promotion generally and health education specifically.

Cycle of change

Prochaska and DiClemente's now famous cycle of change[8] identifies five stages: pre-contemplation, contemplation, planning, action and relapse. Individuals must move through each stage before change is internalised and accustomed (figure 8.1). The model identifies five stages of change and argues that change is not an 'either/or' thing but that people gradually progress though these stages.

Stage 1: Pre-contemplative – unwilling to change and happy with lifestyle. Not receptive to interference. ('You've got to die sometime.')

Stage 2: Contemplative – thinking about changing but not just now. Receptive to information. ('I'd love to change but I just feel I can't.')

Stage 3: Planning – a timeframe for change exists. ('I'm going to change my eating habits at my next birthday.')

Stage 4: Action – taking steps to change. They are taking more exercise, eating fewer calories.

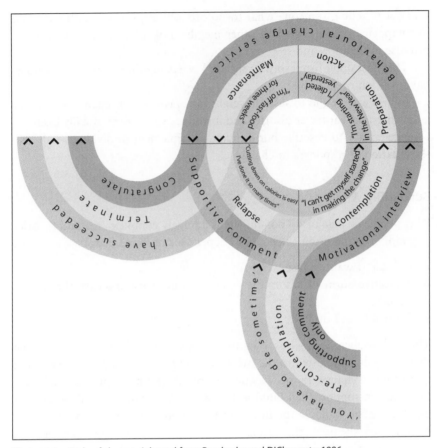

Figure 8.1 Cycle of change. Adapted from Prochaska and DiClemente, 1986.

Stage 5: Relapse – failed to maintain change and have gone back to their old ways, mainly to pre-contemplative stage.

They may cycle through these stages a number of times before change is successful.

Cognitive dissonance

People are more likely to change – move through the five stages of change – if empowered to do so. Empowerment is not something a pharmacist or general practitioner can give someone; empowerment is internal to the individual. The patient 'is' empowered rather than 'was' empowered. Cognitive dissonance describes the likelihood of an individual changing. In simple terms, cognitive dissonance measures the difference between what a person does (the behaviour) and what the person knows (cognitive) they should be doing. This difference is cognitive dissonance and the bigger this difference, the more likely change will occur in an attempt to resolve this internal conflict.

Cognitive dissonance can be created in a number of ways. Having a heart attack will increase cognitive dissonance with a smoking behaviour. A television advertisement on the carnage caused by drinking and driving will increase cognitive dissonance in the person who drives home from the party after a few glasses of wine. Healthcare professionals can be effective in creating cognitive dissonance by raising and discussing the behaviour in a non-threatening and non-judgemental way. But, done incorrectly, these discussions only serve to create resistance to change as the patient attempts to justify the behaviour internally. We all do it. Faced with an authority figure (the pharmacist or general practitioner) who complains about our behaviour (eating too much fatty food) we find the need to argue our case: 'I don't drink or smoke so why are you picking on me about my eating?'; 'Surely some fats are good for you.'

When we defend ourselves, we endorse our behaviours; this is resistance and makes further change less likely. ('When I hear myself talk I learn who I am.'[9])

Pharmacists wishing to support communities and individuals not to become obese and to reduce weight in those who are obese need to develop an understanding of the cycle of change and the additional techniques that will support movement through each stage. 'Change talk' refers to the discussions where the benefits of change are endorsed. Encouraging as much change talk as possible is a key to supporting effective change. Change talk is the opposite to resistance to change. To create change talk it is important for the healthcare practitioner to focus the client on discussing:

- the disadvantage of the status quo ('When I see myself in the mirror I just look terrible.')
- the advantages of the new future that includes the change ('I'm really going to enjoy getting into all those dresses that don't fit me now').

Assessing the individual's readiness to manage the target behaviours and then use stage-specific skills to motivate change and help the patient to move into the next stage of readiness is key to implementing a successful behaviour-based obesity management service. People who are pre-contemplative will be spurred to contemplation when they have internalised sufficient objective information that creates cognitive dissonance and pushes them on.

People are more likely to change when the decision is theirs. The healthcare professional cannot control, motivate or save the patient but they can provide sufficient and understandable information in a caring, trusting context in which people feel safe and comfortable to discuss problems and successes. Lecturing and blaming are counterproductive.

If people do not know what to do or how to do it, or if they believe they do not have the skills or resources to do what is necessary, then change will not occur. Interventions that will help people understand what is needed help people change.

Motivational interviewing technique

Motivational interviewing technique (MIT) as a complementary process to the cycle of change was first targeted at people with addictive behaviours, but now is used to assist healthcare professionals in managing patients with a range of needs, including obesity.[10] It is a strategy to help patients make a commitment to change. The purpose of MIT is to help people overcome ambivalence towards change. People may believe that the change is not truly necessary or they may not understand the seriousness of the condition. Ambivalence affects a person's readiness to change. It is the reason we do not change when we know we should but we have as many reasons for sticking with a behaviour as we have for changing and so we stick with the behaviour; it's a default option.

MIT presents the healthcare professional with an empathetic style of working with people, which supports that person in what is often a difficult behavioural change. It is a person-centred yet directive approach that can be learned through acquiring and integrating a set of principles and skills.

It creates cognitive dissonance without making the patient feel threatened or pressured. Change creates fear and anxiety in all of us and this results in ambivalence – not being sure of what to do. Inevitably we stay where we are; we fail to change. When faced with a need to change, people weigh up the pros and cons. Ambivalence is often the result of a poorly reasoned internal debate – where the need for change is insufficiently strong and ambivalence wins. We stay where we are. 'Faced with the choice between changing one's mind and proving that there is no need to do so, almost everyone gets busy on the proof.' (John Kenneth Galbraith).

Ambivalence is the enemy of change. It will postpone change, sometimes indefinitely. Successful change involves realising that change is needed and believing that change can be successful. MIT is used at any of the stages of change but is possibly most effective at stage 2 – contemplation – those individuals who know they should change but need encouragement to plan (stage 3) and take action (stage 4).

MIT is based on a philosophy that can be broken down into six elements:

- *Client resistance to change is typically a behaviour evoked by environmental conditions.* After the Vietnam War, America planned for a huge heroin abuse problem within the veterans' population; however, this did not happen. The environment that supported the use and abuse of heroin was not present when veterans returned to the family unit.

- *The client/counsellor relationship should be collaborative and friendly.* Positive reinforcement is key to getting someone to focus on long-term goals rather than continue to focus on short-term gains at the cost of long-term goals. In a collaborative environment, clients are more likely to open up.
- *Motivational interviewing gives priority to resolving ambivalence.* Too often counsellors put emphasis on change rather than consideration of the issues that will cause relapse when a change strategy is implemented.
- *The counsellor does not prescribe specific methods or techniques.* You can certainly educate clients on the options but the choice of what option is taken must be the client's. Ultimately it is for the client to choose his/her behaviour.
- *Clients are responsible for their progress.* The counsellor cannot assume this responsibility.
- *MIT focuses on the client's sense of self-efficacy.* The client must be able to feel that he/she can make a successful change in their lives.

Five principles underpin MIT:

- *Have empathy.* It is easy to be judgemental and impatient with clients but where the patient's views and opinions are respected, and their difficulty with change appreciated, success is more likely. Patients who seem to be unwilling or uncooperative with change are not necessarily being obstructive. This may merely reflect their way of dealing with the situation. We express empathy by asking open-ended questions and using reflective listening skills. The client needs to feel that we understand them.
- *Develop discrepancies.* To eradicate ambivalence, the patient must be motivated towards the desired behaviour. Persuasive strategies can fail miserably for some, since it can cause resistance that acts against change. We all know the frustration of arguing with a committed smoker on the merits of stopping. Through use of open questions, the pharmacist will attempt to identify existing discrepancies. In this way, the patient, rather than the pharmacist, will come up with and reinforce the reason for change. Believing ourselves that change is necessary is core to ensuring successful change.
- *Avoid arguing.* MIT is confrontational in its purpose. It must increase an individual's awareness of the problem and the need to change. This differs from argument, where there is an attempt to persuade the patient that they have a problem when that patient is unwilling or unready to accept it. Arguing increases resistance.

- *Roll with resistance.* Trying to convince patients who need to change but are resistant to doing so causes frustration. Resistance should be identified ('I really don't like eating these types of foods'), and an attempt to solve the problem perhaps by providing more information. You might, for example, suggest alternative, more palatable foods.
- *Support self-efficacy.* A key problem to successful change is the patient's lack of belief that they can succeed. When you are 22 stones getting to 18 stones is a major feat. Positive reinforcement is vital. This is done by praising small gains, by endorsing their efforts and by providing clarification of what they are doing.

Practice

In practice, the essence of MIT is given in the mnemonic OARS: open-ended questions, affirmations, reflective listening and summaries. The following is a question sequence used in MIT. It is important that, once a question is asked, the pharmacist does not offer solutions. This can be very difficult for practitioners trained to give advice. The purpose of MIT is to allow the patient to come up with their own solutions to their own problems. The pharmacist might ask these questions over a period of weeks – each time the patient visits the pharmacy perhaps.

Question 1: 'Tell me about the good things and the less good things about . . .'

The patient explores the positive things about the behaviour and then the negative things about it. In MIT, negative words like 'bad things' are not used. This is to avoid labelling behaviours in a judgemental way. Labelling increases resistance. Listening skills are essential. Advice must not be given but clarification can be sought by using probing questions. Let the patient discuss the issue in a supportive and respectful environment. In this way rapport will be built and will make suggestions made later in the interview more effective.

Question 2: 'Tell me about a typical day in relation to . . .'

The patient is offered the opportunity to describe what a typical day is like, for example, by describing their diet. The patient can list what they eat over a typical 24-hour period, and this will provide information that can be acted upon later – avoid the desire to give advice or to offer solutions at this time. Again the process is to allow the patient, in a supportive and non-judgemental environment, to more fully appreciate what they are doing. Use of probing questions will further elucidate information and add to the patient's 'learning' about themselves.

Question 3: 'What would you like to achieve?'

Again at this stage solutions are not offered. Probing questions are used to further clarify the patient's priorities. ('I would like to lose *all* this weight but feel that if I were able to get to 18 stones, I would be very pleased with myself.') This type of declaration identifies a more achievable goal than, say, getting to 12 stones – a target body mass index.

Question 4: 'What do you need to know from me?'

Information is offered to allow the patient to understand the health risk better, and the solutions to reducing that risk. They may want more information on what types and how much fat they should include in their diet. Information provided should be correct, objective and non-judgemental. It should be provided to allow patients to motivate them towards change. At this stage the pharmacist is, for the first time, addressing solutions. Options for support can be considered, such as outlining the available weight-loss diets, local support group, pharmacy or general practitioner based services and pharmacological agents available.

Question 5: 'So what are you going to do?'

In the previous questions, the patient has been steered gently to a change attempt. In addition they will have been motivated to feel that this change is possible. It is better if a number of options exist so that the patient can make his or her choice. We are all more likely to comply when the choice has been ours.

Case study

The following is a discussion between the pharmacist and a woman who has been asking about an over-the-counter weight-loss product that is sold in the pharmacy. The pharmacist uses this opportunity to initiate a brief intervention. Where appropriate, the pharmacist's interventions are identified as open questioning, affirmations, reflective listening or summaries (OARS), and the patient's behaviours are labelled as 'change talk' or 'resistance'.

Patient: 'Are these slimming-aid capsules any good?'
Pharmacist: 'I suppose it depends on what you mean by "good". What are you trying to achieve?' (Open question)
Patient: 'I am always trying to lose weight but it never seems to work for me. I'm big boned, you see, and nothing seems to work for me.' (Resistance and lack of self-efficacy)
Pharmacist: 'Tell me about the different methods of losing weight you have already tried.' (Open question)

Patient: 'I used the Atkins Diet for 3 months, lost nearly 2 stones and then put it all back on again. I lost a stone last summer on the South Beach Diet but it's all back on again. Nothing seems to work for me.' (Resistance)

Pharmacist: 'So you've tried a number of the popular diets to lose weight and whereas they worked at the time, when you stopped using the diet you eventually put the weight back on again.' (Summaries/ reflective listening)

Patient: 'I just can't seem to stick to the diets for very long. I suppose I should just be happy with the way I am.' (Resistance)

Pharmacist: 'Losing weight will make you feel better about yourself but it will also greatly improve your quality of life and reduce your risk of disease.' (Affirmation)

Patient: 'I've been so fat for so long it won't really matter at this stage.' (Resistance)

Pharmacist: 'Tell me about a typical day regarding your eating pattern and about what activity or exercise you get.' (Open question)

The woman describes her diet and activity pattern as follows:

Morning
- eats very little, perhaps tea with a slice of toast with butter.
- mid-morning snack – three biscuits (chocolate)
- activity – goes to the shops at the corner. On Tuesdays, goes to the social security office by taxi. On Sundays, goes to friends' house.

Morning/afternoon 11.00 a.m.–1.00 p.m.
- meal – eats a sandwich (ham and cheese) with chips
- snacks – Coke and crisps
- activity – watches television.

Afternoon 1.00–3.00 p.m.
- meal: nothing
- snack: crisps and Coke
- activity: might go to the shops for cigarettes and to visit off-licence

Afternoon 3.00–6.00 p.m.
- meal: meat or chicken, vegetables (carrots or cabbage) and potatoes with butter
- snack: none

Evening 6.00–11.00 p.m.

- meal: none
- snack: chocolate, crisps and Coke, three glasses of wine
- activity: seldom goes out as she believes the estate is not safe.

Pharmacist: 'From what you have just told me, which foods in your diet do you think are healthy foods and which foods are unhealthy' (Open question)

Patient: 'I know the sweets, crisps and Coke drinks are the unhealthy foods.'

Pharmacist: 'You're right, you are eating about 1000 calories a day in unhealthy snacks.'

Patient: 'Yeah, if I were to cut out even half of these then I could lose a bit of weight at least.' (Change talk)

Pharmacist: 'About one or two pounds in a week in fact.' (Affirmation)

Patient: 'Over 6 months, that might give me over a stone in weight loss.' (Change talk)

Pharmacist: 'Add to this an increased amount of moderate exercise and you could really improve your weight problem in a short period of time. If you want, I can get more information for you the next time you're in.'

In this conversation a lot of information was generated by the use of open-ended questions that provide a basis for the pharmacist to begin gently to support an outline plan to address this individual's weight management problem. Above all, this MIT discussion was supportive and non-confrontational. The conversation was shifted from the initially negative resistance-type talk to more change talk. This conversation has highlighted that the woman's solution to her weight problem lies with her poor diet, in particular, her high level of snacking and also in her lack of exercise. She has been given options to think about but has not been told what to do.

Cognitive behavioural therapy

Cognitive behavioural therapy (CBT) is a term that covers a number of therapies designed to help people solve problems and is mainly targeted at anxiety, depression, drug misuse, or post-traumatic stress disorder but has also been found to be effective in eating disorders such as anorexia and in binge eating that leads to obesity.

CBT builds on two earlier types of psychotherapy:

- cognitive therapy, designed to change people's thoughts, beliefs, attitudes and expectations
- behavioural therapy (also known as behaviourism), designed to change how people act.

American psychotherapist, Aaron Beck,[12] who was a key figure in the development of CBT, believed that how we think about a situation influences our behaviour. In turn, our behaviour can influence how we think and feel. It is therefore necessary to change both cognition (the act of thinking) and behaviour (what we do) at the same time. This is known as cognitive behavioural therapy.

In short-term studies, cognitive behavioural therapy can induce weight loss of around 10%, but results have not translated as well in the longer term. Behavioural therapy, as one element in an extended programme of long-term support, alongside regular physical activity and nutritional strategies, is much more successful. For example, CBT combined with very low-energy diets has produced significant weight loss in various studies.[13]

Different strands of CBP have been minutely analysed, and a whole encyclopaedia of phrases and descriptions invented, many of which hide simple and effective concepts. These include: self-monitoring, stimulus control, relapse management, social support and challenging negative thinking.[13]

In obesity management, the most basic form of self-monitoring is a food and activity diary: what is eaten, where it was eaten, in what circumstances, and what emotional feelings or triggers may have been involved. It also records levels and circumstances of physical activity. A food diary clarifies eating patterns and behaviours, especially the events that trigger eating and a person's relationship with food, with a view to altering established patterns once they have been identified. Even the fact of being asked to record intake in a diary can often on its own have a dramatic effect on a person's food intake, partly because they may become aware of their own bad habits, seeing them written in black and white, and partly by avoiding certain foods out of embarrassment, in the knowledge that a healthcare professional is going to scrutinise any deviations from the 'straight and narrow'. Once created, the food diary can be used as part of the treatment plan, by monitoring progress towards new dietary goals. Long-term weight management has been shown to improve when food records are used.[14]

Stimulus control

Stimulus control requires a person to recognise the different stimuli that they have to eat, only one of which is feeling physically hungry. Raiding the fridge for cheese on arriving home from work may be more likely to be because of stress than hunger; the stimulus control therefore is remove the cheese – don't buy it, or hide it – or remove the stress. Other 'external cues' for eating not related to hunger include:

- time – it is coffee break, and coffee and biscuits always go together
- the presence of food – eating it because it is there; finishing a plateful because it is rude or wasteful not to
- social cues – everyone else is having biscuits with their coffee, or cheese with their port.

Stimulus control involves avoiding external cues, for instance, taking the route home that avoids passing the fish and chip shop. Controlling eating at the last stage of the process is extremely difficult, for instance, when one is already looking at the price of cod in the fish and chip shop window, able to smell the salt and vinegar, and seeing everyone else coming out of the shop with their meals wrapped in paper. Taking action earlier in the chain of events is much more likely to succeed when the chip supper is a distant proposition, and much less tangible: take a different route home, get off the bus at the stop after the chip shop, not before. Former UK prime minister Margaret Thatcher got into trouble by suggesting that people on low incomes could save money by avoiding shopping when they were hungry; she may have chosen her moment badly but she was merely advocating stimulus control. Other stimuli such as stress or emotional eating can be described as 'internal cues'.

Learned self-control

Learned self-control becomes important when there is no alternative than to pass the chip shop on the way home, or alternatively a rival burger bar opens up on the only other possible route. External temptations become unavoidable, so learned self-control becomes crucial; prolonged repetition of the stimulus to eat is inevitable, but must be resisted. Once enough journeys have been undertaken without a fast-food purchase, the conditioned response will reduce.

'Stress management' is self-explanatory; comfort foods and emotional eating are well recognised as causes of overeating and weight gain in susceptible individuals, although stress may of course, lead to reduction of appetite.

Conclusion

Where the cycle of change provides a theoretical framework to describe how individuals bring about internal behavioural change, both motivational interviewing and cognitive behavioural therapy provide powerful tools for effecting lifestyle change and should be essential skills for all healthcare professionals. However, these can be difficult skills to develop, as most professionals, mainly because of previous experience, find these approaches difficult to incorporate into day-to-day practice and for this reason alone they are often ignored. However, by taking the first steps and beginning to use them practically, by incorporating them in practice and applying them to real patients, then their value and effectiveness will quickly become apparent.

References

1. Winston R. *The Human Mind and How to Make the Most of It*. London: Bantam Press, 2003.
2. Greenfield S. *Brain Story: unlocking our inner world of emotions, memories, ideas and desires*. London: BBC, 2000.
3. West R. *Theory of Addiction*. Oxford: Blackwell, 2006.
4. Pharmacy HealthLink. *Brief Advice*. London: Pharmacy Health Link, 2008.
5. Department of Health. *Choosing Health: making healthier choices easier*. London: Department of Health, 2004.
6. Department of Health. *Our Health, Our Care, Our Say*. London: Department of Health, 2006.
7. Department of Health. *Choosing Health Through Pharmacy: a programme for pharmaceutical public health 2005–2015*. London: Department of Health, 2007.
8. Prochaska J *et al*. Predicting change in smoking status for self-changers. *Addict Behav* 1985; 10: 395–406.
9. Prochaska J, DiClemente C. Stages and processes of self-change of smoking: Towards an integrative model of change. *J Consult Clin Psychol* 1983; 51: 390–395.
10. Miller W, Rollnick S. *Motivational Interviewing: preparing people for change*, 2nd edn. New York: Guilford Press, 2002.
11. Maguire T. *Mind Your Own Business*. Tunbridge Wells: Chemist & Druggist CMP Information, 2003.
12. Beck A. *Cognitive Therapy*, 1971.
13. Rapoport L. Cognitive behaviour therapy in obesity treatment. *Obesity in Practice* 2000; 2: 13–15.
14. Haslam D. *Obesity: your questions answered*. Oxford: Radcliffe Medical Press, 2005.

9

Activity and exercise

A number of years ago a film documentary was televised about two men who, having worked in office jobs for over 30 years, decided to take early retirement and try a new more active career as charcoal burners. The documentary followed them for a few months when they moved from their offices to a cabin deep in the woods. They worked long days felling trees and digging pits to make their charcoal. The film traced their transformation from office workers to manual labourers and, although it was primarily about the change in their quality of life brought about by more physical activity and a more primitive lifestyle, mentally they were much happier and in addition the physical benefits were also quickly evident. Within 3 months each had lost a considerable amount of weight (one over 7.5 kg) yet both claimed they were eating more.

A diet or exercise problem?

In Western societies, research shows that average day-to-day physical activity has declined significantly over the 100 years from 1900 to 2000. Yet this has been a gradual decline over perhaps thousands of years. Our early ancestors spent many hours of each day engaged in moderate or intense physical activity. Hunting and gathering food meant that humans used large amounts of energy in order to survive. As humans became more sophisticated, animals were domesticated and crops planted and this led to an overall reduction in daily energy expenditure needed for securing food. The development of agricultural societies was therefore the first notable decrease in physical activity. The Industrial Revolution, and associated urbanisation, mechanisation and the advent of steam power, is correlated with a further reduction in human energy expenditure. In the 20th century, the dramatic rise in automotive transport reduced the need for walking or cycling, and labour-saving devices, popular with the modern consumer, helped further reduce activity. In addition, work is less and less involved with physical effort compared with that of previous generations.

Of course these societal changes, happening over a few thousand years, have not been associated with genetic changes to human physiology –

genetic changes that might take millions of years to bring about. In relation to our physical activity needs, we have much in common genetically with our hunter-gatherer ancestors yet our lives are lived in very different circumstances, and this is a major cause of, and contributor to, our obesity epidemic.

The food industry, particularly the fast foods and convenience foods industries, have been keen to blame the current population obesity problem on a reduction in energy expenditure through avoidance of exercise rather than from the consumption of too many calories from calorie-dense, highly processed, foods. Vested interest aside, there may be some truth in this, yet to exonerate the fast and convenience foods industries from a role in obesity would be difficult and the protestations of this industry of course merely serves to further confuse the general public on the facts about, and the solutions to, current obesity trends.

What is clear from research, and has been apparent for some years, is that in the energy balance equation, physical activity is every bit as important as nutrition when considering obesity, and it might be even more important in reducing the risk of non-communicable chronic diseases such as diabetes and coronary heart disease.[1]

Physical activity can help to manage and improve many clinical conditions. It can halve the risk of developing coronary heart disease and reduces the risk of developing type 2 diabetes by a similar amount. It has an impact on osteoporosis and various cancers. Being physically active can improve mental health and help people maintain independent living well into their old age.

Colin Waine, a physician with a specialist interest in obesity and its management,[1] strongly endorses the view that a lack of exercise, rather than an increase in calorie intake, is the primary cause of our current obesity problem. The paradox, he claims, is that our obesity epidemic is occurring at a time of reduced food intake and this suggests that levels of energy expenditure have declined more rapidly, specifically from the 1970s to the present, and there is evidence to support this view. Data from national food surveys show that our daily energy intake has declined for a number of decades.[2] One epidemiological study found that individuals who were sedentary at the start of a study period and were followed up for 10 years, were more than twice as likely to experience considerable weight gain compared with study subjects who were active.[3]

Few studies have directly compared dietary interventions with exercise intervention in achieving successful weight loss. In one study, obese subjects were put onto a 700 kcal deficient diet and compared with a second group of obese subjects who walked on a treadmill for 60 minutes per day. Both groups lost 7.5 kg over the 12 weeks of the study but the exercise group lost more body fat while the diet group had greater loss of muscle mass. Given the importance of muscle mass in determining basic metabolic rate, the authors concluded that exercise was overall the most effective intervention.[4]

It has been known for some time that even a small daily imbalance in energy intake can result, over a decade, in a considerable weight gain. From national surveys, it has been shown that English activity patterns have fallen in recent decades and, even though overall dietary calories have also fallen, there is an average net gain of 15 kcal per day. Over a week this is over 100 kcal; in a month it is 400 kcal; in a year, 4800 kcal; in 10 years, 48 000 kcal, all of which can translate into an increase in weight of approximately 1 stone (6.3 kg). For those who are obese and wish to achieve significant weight loss, research indicates that they should gradually increase their level of physical activity to expend in excess of 2000 kcal per week.[4] In most individuals this requires between 200 and 300 minutes of exercise per week or 30–45 minutes per day. Ideally most of this activity should be moderate intensity (55–70% of maximum heart rate) with evidence suggesting that a small amount of this time should be more vigorous activity (over 70% of maximum heart rate).

Exercise patterns

Excessive weight gain is linked to reduced activity more than it is correlated to increased energy intake. It has been established that physically active individuals who eat more than others often weight the least and maintain the highest fitness levels.[4]

In children aged 4–6 years whose food intake is normal but daily energy expenditure averages 25% below the physical activity recommendation, obesity occurs, making a lack of exercise the primary cause of childhood obesity. In the US, 50% of boys and 75% of girls fail to engage in even moderate activity three or more times weekly. In America it has been shown that childhood fatness relates directly to the number of hours spent watching television, a consistent marker for inactivity. Watching television for 3 hours per day leads to a doubling of the risk of obesity and a doubling of the risk of developing type 2 diabetes.[5]

The Health Survey for England[6] showed that only a minority of adults (40% of men and 28% of women) were meeting the Chief Medical Officer's physical activity targets. The good news is that they have increased from 1997 (up from 32% and 21% respectively) yet this is still insufficient to reduce the current obesity levels. For UK adults, only about 25% undertake some form of regular exercise and this figure is similar to rates in the USA. This is common to all age groups but the lower social groups tend to take less exercise, again a fact that will have an impact on social inequalities in health.

A British Heart Foundation survey[7] in 2007 found that only 38% of the British adult population would be motivated to do more exercise if their life depended on it. Exercise, it seems, is something many people are unwilling to engage in.

Outside the UK and the US, activity levels in the populations of most industrialised countries have also been falling significantly over the past 50 years.[1] Where approximately only 25% of Americans report exercising regularly, even these individuals find compliance difficult with other obligations, particularly changing priorities and variable motivation, regularly causing disruption in the amount of exercise undertaken. There is a considerable challenge for national governments in bringing about an increase in national physical activity levels. Firstly it requires that the consequences of being physically inactive be understood as well as the benefits of increased activity being promoted.

The environment and obesity

Inactivity has its roots in our physical environmental. Modern society goes to great lengths to facilitate the individual in reducing daily energy output. Elevators, escalators and automatic doors assist us in transiting modern buildings without much energy being expended and our leisure time is mostly spent in energy-efficient activities such as watching television or videos and play computer games that only require a rapid thumb movement. Indeed the modern human environment has been designed in such a way that getting more active can prove challenging.

The 'default option', discussed in previous chapters, has a huge impact on the types of choices people make in their environments. For example, exiting an underground station and given the option between taking an escalator or lift and walking up the stairs, passengers are more likely to choose the former. Removing the escalator makes the stairs the default option, and in this case ensures that getting from the platform to ground level is achieved with a greater expenditure of energy. In practice this is difficult, since disability access in public places is an important issue and the law must be observed. Yet there is a certain irony in that in ensuring access for the disabled, we are possibly conspiring to increase their number. Architects of new buildings are designing buildings where the default option requires less and less effort – certainly lifts to upper floors are generally more visible than staircases, so that even those choosing to walk up the stairs find it difficult to locate them.

To address this problem, the National Institute for Health and Clinical Excellence (NICE) guidance on creating built environments that help people become more physically active was published in 2008.[8] Since the built environment has been identified as a major contributor to the development of obesity, action needs to be taken to encourage people to take the option that expends more energy. Town planners, designers and architects all have a key responsibility in ensuring that the spaces and buildings they are responsible for producing offer those who use their creations the possibility of expending energy that will maintain and improve health. Above all, we need to assist people to be more physically active, providing better walking and cycling routes, and building offices and homes with better access and signposting to stairs.

Why activity matters

Human metabolism, like everything else in the universe, adheres to the second law of thermodynamics and, since energy cannot be created or destroyed, energy expenditure through physical activity becomes one side of the 'energy-in–energy-out' equation and therefore an unchecked and long-term decrease in physical activity with maintenance of calorie intake will logically result in obesity (figure 9.1).

Physical activity has considerable influence on body composition, particularly fat content, lean tissue mass and bone density. Physical activity shares a common metabolic pathway with nutrition and as a result can offset some of the risks associated with consumptions of certain foods. Keeping physically active can help reduce the risk of coronary heart disease (CHD), type 2 diabetes and joint problems. Sustained regular physical activity will reduce weight, reduce total cholesterol and raise high-density lipoprotein cholesterol. In addition, it will improve cardiovascular fitness, which will increase the chances of survival should a heart attack occur.

Evidence from a number of studies over the past 50 years identifies the increased risk of CHD in unfit people. The most notable of these studies, initiated in the 1970s, looked at post office workers and showed that those with desk jobs had a much greater risk of myocardial infarction than those delivering letters.[9]

More recent studies underpin the benefits of increased exercise in reducing the incidence of type 2 diabetes. In a Finnish study, exercise brought about a reduction in body weight and an overall reduction in the

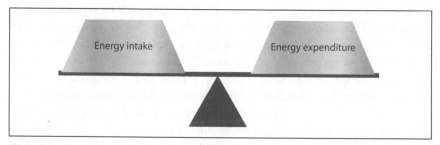

Figure 9.1 The energy balance. To keep weight steady, energy intake must be equal to energy expenditure.

risk of developing type 2 diabetes by between 11% and 23%.[10] In addition, an American study that involved taking 30 minutes of moderate exercise per day in combination with a low-fat diet, gave a 5–8% drop in body weight but a 20% reduction in the risk of developing type 2 diabetes.[11]

Exercise is good and, it seems, more exercise is better still. Government guidelines for the UK[12] recommend that adults should engage in a minimum of 30 minutes of at least moderate-intensity physical activity on five or more days of the week.

As we have seen, few people comply with this recommendation and this might be that individuals view daily exercise as difficult to build into a busy lifestyle – yet it must be remembered that this amount of exercise will not reduce body weight – at best it will only halt weight gain. More exercise is required to reduce weight and of course this should ideally be done in conjunction with a calorie-reduced diet.

Exercise physiology

At a cellular level, energy is provided by molecules of adenosine triphosphate (ATP) and ATP must be available in the cell to allow normal metabolic function to continue. In the body, a number of methods have evolved that ensures ATP is always available. Our cells can break down glucose anaerobically to produce ATP by fermentation, a primitive cellular process whereby ATP is produced without oxygen but this is not normally a significant contributor to cellular ATP. More commonly, our cells use respiration, the oxygen-based aerobic intracellular process, to produce ATP. Respiration occurs in the mitochondria, where glucose and fats, and sometimes proteins after deamination, are oxidised to produce ATP that is then used for energy such as allowing muscles to move, nerve impulses to fire and metabolic processes to function.

Misconceptions about exercise

Perhaps many people fail to engage in regular exercise or planned activity because of misconceptions about the role of exercise in body weight management. Many believe exercise stimulates appetite that in turn encourages more calories to be consumed than has been expended during the exercise. In addition, many believe that the small calorie-burning effect of normal exercise does not expend sufficient energy to have any meaningful impact on body weight. They assume that only a punishing amount of exercise will shift a small amount of body weight. Perhaps they have looked at the charts and calculated that a specific amount of activity will take many hours to produce a useful gain. For example, to lose 1 pound (0.45 kg) of fat will require 10 hours of chopping wood. But regular activity quickly adds up and the gain is appreciated over a period of months. Weight has taken years to accumulate and therefore it is reasonable to assume that weight loss cannot happen overnight but rather, with sustained effort, will happen over a number of months.

Individuals involved in regular moderate exercise are much better at regulating energy intake and matching it to daily energy expenditure. Individuals who fail to take any exercise are incapable of matching energy intake and expenditure and therefore are more likely to eat too many calories and as a result put on weight. Those with highly active lifestyles, such as the charcoal burners in the introduction to this chapter, consume about twice as many calories as sedentary workers but have less body fat. Similarly endurance athletes such as marathon runners, cross-country skiers and cyclists will consume 4000 kcal daily or more yet are the leanest in the population. The Olympic gold-medal winning swimmer Michael Phelps was estimated to consume over 7000 calories per day when he was winning his 14 gold medals in Beijing in 2008.

The small compensatory appetite-stimulating effect associated with moderate activity is offset by the energy expenditure associated with the activity. Research has shown that over a 16-month period, overweight people who began exercising did not increase the amounts of carbohydrates, fat or protein they consumed but they did lose weight.

A small amount of exercise weekly, such as five 30-minute sessions that raise pulse rate and increase the rate of breathing will make a difference. Moderate-intensity activity will:

- improve circulation
- improve the efficiency of heart and lungs
- help reduce stress
- help keep bones healthy (in women it will protect against osteoporosis after the menopause)
- help individuals to stay active at work and play for longer.

Tangible benefits of regular exercise include making people more proud of their bodies, and they sleep better. This aside, it is now clear that government targets for exercise and activity, particularly in the UK, may be inadequate as the more exercise that you take the better the benefits. The current guidelines perhaps should be seen as a minimum requirement and once activity programmes are initiated, clients should be encouraged to up their exercise with a view to making greater health gains. Regular exercise produces less accumulation of the central adipose tissue that is associated with ageing and an increased risk of CHD and type 2 diabetes. In practical terms, this can be difficult for many – especially those overweight and over 50 years of age. Obese people can find exercise difficult and care must be taken to ensure that they do not injure themselves when becoming involved in strenuous exercise.

Often it is best, when discussing exercise with overweight and obese people, to use the word 'activity', since exercise has a connotation of formalised action that many may feel they are unable to comply with. Listening to clients and finding out their personal barriers to taking exercise is a useful way to start supporting them towards change. For example, they might not be happy walking in their neighbourhood at night – walking with a few friends might be the way to resolve this.

What activity?

It is vital that exercise and activity are not seen as exclusively linked to organised exercise sessions such as attending a gym or in organised sporting activity. These are excellent ways of obtaining exercise, and commercial gyms for some people may be a suitable way of losing weight, yet there is little evidence to show the efficacy of gyms – in fact, there is evidence to the contrary. It has been claimed that the mushrooming of private gyms fails to address the obesity epidemic.[13] This research, which focused on the US where health clubs have been a commercial success for years yet obesity levels have also risen, found that half of health club members were in the top 20% of income earners; at the very bottom, excluded from this market, were those individuals most likely to be inactive and as a result obese. The conclusion was that gyms promoted exercise as something to be squeezed into the daily routine, and that the focus was on enhanced body image rather than on improved health.

Exercise and activity should be promoted in whatever way is most convenient to the individual. Of course it is important to advise clients to start gently and work up slowly. To ensure individuals will continue with the exercise, they should be encouraged to choose an activity that they enjoy and which is compatible with their physical condition. If they do so, they are more likely to continue and gain benefit. Pharmacist and other primary

Table 9.1 Activities related to energy expended over time

Activity	Time	Energy (kcals)
Reading aloud	30 minutes	15
Washing dishes	15 minutes	19
Bicycle riding	60 minutes	150
Playing squash	60 minutes	916
Running	50 minutes	660
Walking	60 minutes	400

care workers can also play a key role in advising parents to encourage their children to take part in exercise so that this will become a lifelong habit. Table 9.1 links common daily activities and the energy expended in undertaking them.

Fitness

There are three elements to getting fit: stamina, suppleness and strength. Different exercises work on each element of fitness and to a different degree – for example, jogging improves stamina but does little for strength while yoga improves suppleness but does nothing for stamina. Table 9.2 gives an indication of the main elements of fitness derived from an exercise type.

Strength: the strength of muscles is increased when they are pushed against a resistance. If we do not constantly strengthen our muscles, we lose the ability to lift and carry things and posture suffers since the muscles that support the body will weaken.

Suppleness: this is the ease with which the joints can be flexed without causing damage. Through inactivity, muscles and joints get stiff, restricting bending and stretching. Joints must be moved through the full range of movements possible, but without overdoing it.

Stamina: This is a measure of the ability to carry on an exercise after the first 5 minutes or so. This relates to the ability of the body to use oxygen in the exercise process, i.e. aerobic fitness. People who are unfit are unable to use oxygen easily to create energy. Stamina training allows more deep breathing, the heart pumps oxygenated blood to muscles more efficiently and muscles are more efficient at utilising oxygen. As stamina improves, exercise can go on for longer and there is less breathlessness.

Monitoring fitness

Pulse rate is a simple, accurate and convenient monitor of fitness. A baseline value can be obtained first thing in the morning before eating or drinking.

Table 9.2 Elements of fitness

Fitness element	Initial activities	Activities once fit
Strength	Swimming, digging the garden, hill walking	Circuit training, press ups, weight training
Suppleness	Warm-up and stretches, walking and swimming	Yoga, aerobics/keep fit, squash
Stamina	Swimming, walking, cycling	Aerobic exercise, jogging, circuit training, rowing

Find the pulse with the index finger and count the pulses for 60 seconds (the result is therefore in beats per minute, or bpm). Resting pulse rate (RestPR) is higher in those who are unfit, typically above 70 bpm. When an individual is fit, the RestPR will generally be below 70; athletes at the peak of their fitness could have a RestPR of around 40 bpm.

Pulse rate after taking a prescribed amount of moderate exercise is termed the exercise pulse rate (EPR) and the pulse rate 1 minute after stopping exercising is termed the recovery pulse rate (RecPR). Using these three values, RestPR, EPR and RecPR, provides a simple way of advising an individual about their level of fitness and what exercise they should be taking.

The step test

The step test is used to assess an individual's fitness. To perform the step test, use a 20 cm (8 inch) high step; step up, right foot first, onto the step and down again, left food first. This procedure should take 10 seconds and should be repeated for 3 minutes. After 3 minutes stop the exercise and record the EPR. Rest for 1 minute and record the RecRP. As one gets fitter, the RestPR and EPR get lower and the recovery pulse rate gets closer to the resting pulse rate.

To calculate the initial target EPR for an individual, take the maximum pulse rate as 220 bpm, and from this subtract the individual's age in years, then calculate 75% of the answer to give the upper level of the target pulse rate for exercise and 55% for the lower level of 'moderate intensity' exercise. This is the pulse rate an individual should aim to achieve initially and to maintain this for 30 minutes. As the individual becomes fitter, the exercise level can be and should be increased. For example, for a 50-year-old man, the upper level target pulse rate is:

220 (maximum PR) − 50 (years) × 0.75 = 127.5 bpm.

The lower level target pulse rate is:

220 (maximum PR) − 50 (years) × 0.55 = 93.5 beats per minute.

For this individual an exercise regimen, such as walking or gentle jogging, which raises pulse rate to between 95 and 125 bpm and should be recommended to be maintained for 30 minutes. As the individual become fitter, the exercise will need to be increased to achieve this target exercise pulse rate. For this individual, exercise that produces a EPR of greater than 127 bpm would be classified as 'vigorous activity'.

Another way of estimating how to comply with exercise guidelines is to take sufficient physical activity to elevate total energy expenditure to 160–180% of resting metabolic rate.[14] One method of achieving this goal is by walking 60–90 minutes every day but this type of commitment is difficult to achieve and sustain for most. If pulse rate is used as a proxy for resting metabolic rate then the average resting pulse rate of 70 bpm would need to be increased to 112–126 bpm.

Current guidelines on physical activity are aimed at promoting physical activity among the sedentary. However, the benefits of this may be limited unless activity is maintained consistently without extended interruption.

Case study

One of the authors, TM, once a sedentary academic type, took up jogging on a running machine at a local gym. Initially his resting pulse rate was 75 bpm and his starting exercise programme was jogging for 20 minutes at a speed of 9 km/hour, achieving an EPR of 120 bpm at the end of this exercise period. This programme continued for 1 month, then he increased the running machine speed to 10 km/hour for 20 minutes and then in month 3 he increased the speed to 11 km/hour, still for 20 minutes. At this speed, the EPR was 138 bpm at the end of the exercise period and his RecPR was 128 bpm.

At month 6 he began to run for a longer time at each session, completing 10 km (55 minutes at 11 km/hour) and doing this twice weekly for a further 3 months. At the end of each run his EPR was 155 bpm, his RecPR was 125 bpm and his RestPR was now 65 bpm. When he started out on this exercise programme, his weight was 83 kg and over the 9 months of this exercise programme, his weight fell to 77 kg – a loss of 6 kg in 9 months, during which time he did not modify his eating habits in any way.

Avoiding injury

Patients should be instructed not to exercise if they feel ill, e.g. have flu or a common cold. Exercise should not be started until 1 hour after food, should never be taken under the influence of alcohol or in extreme heat or cold. Exercise should be stopped if the individual experiences chest or leg pain or becomes uncomfortably breathless, feels dizzy or faint or breaks out in a cold sweat.

Individuals should be fit enough for the exercise they are undertaking. Proper clothing, particularly footwear, is essential to avoid injury. Limbering or warming up is important. All the muscles to be used should first be stretched. The first 5 minutes should be the warm-up period, followed by 20 minutes of hard work and the final 5 minutes working more slowly.

The UK Chief Medical Officer stated that the people who will benefit most from physical activity are inactive people who begin to take part in regular moderate-intensity activity. If these people increase their level of activity gradually, they are unlikely to face undue risks.[15]

Keep it up

The good news is that an increase in exercise can effectively contribute to controlling weight gain and can, when of sufficient regularity and intensity, contribute to weight loss. It works both ways, however, and a decrease in physical activity results in weight gain. What has not been so clear is whether the magnitudes of these changes in weight are equal. Unequal (asymmetric) weight changes could contribute to overall weight gain or loss among individuals with seasonal or irregular activity.

In one study,[16] changes in adiposity were compared with the running distances at baseline and follow up in men and women who reported exercise increase and these were compared with a group of men and women in whom exercise decreased. The study involved 7.7 years of follow up. The findings showed that where running decreased, there was a significant gain in weight and unless the individual, when running was resumed, ran more than 32 km a week, it was unlikely that the weight gain, a result of stopping the exercise, would be offset by the renewed running regime. The implications are clear; exercise in relation to weight gain is asymmetrical; it can prove difficult to remove fat gained from a period of inactivity when exercise is resumed. Keeping up the exercise is vital if weight gain is to be avoided.

How do we keep it up?

Few will be able to commit to visiting a gym regularly as a means of taking more exercise. Indeed many will feel intimidated in such an environment and will prefer to seek out other ways of getting their exercise. In this way activity is often a better and acceptable term than exercise. Daily chores such as gardening and cleaning the house can meaningfully contribute to an overall daily energy output. Suggested activity is provided in box 9.1.

The Government says

NICE Guidance issued in 2006[17] stresses that primary care practitioners should take the opportunity whenever possible, to identify inactive adults and advise them to be more active. Moderate physical activity is equivalent to brisk walking (around 8 km/hour or 5 miles/hour) but includes not just sports or formal exercise, but day-to-day activity too.

Research suggests that the 30 minutes does not have to be taken in one go – it can be built up in bouts of 10 minutes or more, making it easier to achieve, especially for older people. But to prevent obesity in the absence of a reduction in energy intake, many people may need 45–60 minutes of moderate activity each day. To prevent regaining weight following weight

> *Box 9.1* Examples of moderate-intensity activity (after ref. 17)
>
> - brisk walking
> - cycling
> - swimming (with moderate effort)
> - stair climbing (with moderate effort)
> - gardening – digging, pushing mower or sweeping leaves
> - general house cleaning
> - painting and decorating
> - general callisthenics (sit-ups, push-ups, chin-ups)
> - gentle racquet sports such as table tennis and badminton (social)
> - golf – walking, wheeling or carrying clubs

loss among people who have been obese, 60–90 minutes of moderate activity per day may be needed.

For children and young people, the facts are less clear on the amount of activity required. They should achieve a total of at least 60 minutes of at least moderate-intensity physical activity daily yet this may be inadequate to prevent the development of obesity. Only about 70% of children meet the current recommendations yet the prevalence of obesity continues to rise. Children should be given the opportunity and support to do more regular, structured physical activity, such as football, swimming or dancing. The choice of activity should be made with the child, and be appropriate to their ability and confidence.

The definition of moderate-intensity physical activity varies according to the fitness level of the individual.[18] A person doing moderate-intensity activity will usually experience an increase in breathing rate, an increase in heart rate and a feeling of increased warmth. Ideally primary healthcare workers should become involved in:

- brief interventions in primary care
- exercise referral schemes
- pedometer supply
- community-based exercise programmes (for walking and cycling).

Using pedometers to guide physical activity, even when not accompanied by dietary interventions, promotes modest weight loss among sedentary and obese or overweight individuals.[19]

References

1. Waine C. *Obesity and Weight Management in Primary Care* Oxford: Blackwell Science, 2003.
2. Prentice A M, Jebb S A. Obesity in Britain; gluttony or sloth? *BMJ* 1995; 311: 437–439.

3. Paffenbarger R S *et al*. The association of changes in physical activity level and other lifestyle characteristics with mortality among men. *New Engl J Med* 1993; 328: 538–545.

4. Ross R *et al*. Reduction in obesity and related co-morbid conditions after diet-induced weight loss or exercise-induced weigh loss in men; a randomised controlled trial. *Ann Intern Med* 2001; 133: 92–103.

5. Centre for Longitudinal Studies. National Child Development Study 2008. http://www.cls.ioe.ac.uk (accessed Feb 2009).

6. NHS Information Centre. *Health Survey for England 2006. Latest trends.* London: National Centre for Social Research, 2008.

7. British Heart Foundation. Statistical website. http://www.heartstats.org (accessed Feb 2009).

8. National Institute for Health and Clinical Excellence. *Workplace Health Promotion: how to encourage employees to be physically active.* London: NICE, May 2008.

9. Bosma H *et al*. Low job control and risk of coronary heart disease in Whitehall II (prospective cohort) study. *BMJ* 1997; 314: 558–565.

10. Tuomilehto J *et al*. Prevention of type 2 diabetes mellitus by changes in lifestyle among subjects with impaired glucose tolerance. *N Engl J Med* 2001; 344: 1343–1350.

11. Carey V J *et al*. Body fat distribution and risk of non-insulin dependent diabetes mellitus in women. The Nurses' Health Study. *Am J Epidemiol* 1997; 145: 614–619.

12. Change4Life. http://www.nhs.uk/change4life (accessed Feb 2009).

13. Smith-Maguire J. Private gyms won't solve fatness crisis (News in brief). *The Times Online*, 7 Nov 2007. www.timesonline.co.uk/tol/news/uk/article2821181.ece (accessed 10 Jul 2009).

14. Erlichman J *et al*. Physical activity and its impact on health outcomes. Paper 2: prevention of unhealthy weight gain and obesity by physical activity: an analysis of the evidence. *Obes Rev* 2002; 3: 273–287.

15. Chief Medical Officer. *Good Doctors, Safer Patients.* London: Department of Health, 2006.

16. Williams T. Asymmetric weight gain and loss from increasing and decreasing exercise. *Med Sci Sports Exerc* 2008; 40: 296–302.

17. National Institute for Health and Clinical Excellence. *Four Commonly Used Methods to Increase Physical Activity.* London: NICE, 2006.

18. Sport England. *Fitness and Exercise Spaces.* Sport England Guidance. http://www.sportengland.org (accessed Feb 2009).

19. Richardson C R *et al*. A meta-analysis of pedometer-based walking interventions and weight loss. *Ann Fam Med* 2008; 6: 69–77.

10

Nutrition and diet

Humans, in common with all living organisms, must consume food to grow and survive and here exists a paradox: although food is essential for life and good health, more food is not necessarily better, yet this is a very difficult concept to quantify and communicate. Unlike cigarette smoking or excessive alcohol intake, which are unnecessary and where public health policy can simply advocate smoking cessation or minimal alcohol consumption, food policy and nutritional guidance tends to be complex, sometimes controversial and often confusing when expressed in public health policy terms.

In generations past, a lack of food was a main cause of disease: malnutrition and specific deficiency diseases were common. Goitre resulted from a lack of iodine, pellagra from a lack of niacin (vitamin B_1) and rickets from a lack of vitamin D. Today, in developed countries, few are malnourished and deficiency diseases are rarely, if ever, seen. In parallel with the ability of Western societies to feed their populations, has come an understanding of the risks associated with the excessive consumption of certain types of foods.

This chapter considers the key components of a healthy diet and how the average modern diet compares with the ideal. Eating sensibly and nutritiously is an important step towards good health. The more balanced and nutritious the diet, the healthier the individual can expect to be. A balanced diet means eating the right amount of foods from all the main food groups; however, most children and adults in the UK do not meet dietary recommendations. Instead a significant proportion of the population, and particularly those on lower incomes, consume less than the recommended amounts of fruit, vegetables and fibre yet more than the recommended amounts of fat, saturated fats, salt and sugar.

With obesity, however, strategies may change. The imposition of the 'balance of good health' may be too late to improve the health, and reduce the risks of someone whose staple nutritional intake has gone badly wrong, resulting in chronic disease. The dietetic care of the obese person is a specialist subject, just as it is in coeliac disease or other malnutrition disorders, and regimes that may be frowned upon in lean individuals such as very low-calorie and low-carbohydrate diets, should be embraced in the management of obesity.[1]

Getting the message

A 'healthy diet' will provide enough food to ensure that the body gets sufficient calories to function optimally, while also providing adequate amounts of minerals and vitamins necessary to construct the enzymes that ensure maintenance of healthy body structures and metabolic systems. In this way health is assured. 'Junk food' is the term used to describe foods that are so highly processed that the vitamin and mineral content has been removed. In addition, processed foods tend to be calorie-dense and high in salt and additives and therefore, if eaten regularly, contribute to obesity and to poor health.

It is not surprising, however, that the public are often confused about what constitutes a 'healthy diet'. Personal preferences for high-sugar, high-fat foods and a cultural predilection for the foods offered to us as children, strongly influence our day-to-day food choices and these preferences are difficult to change. Poor maternal diet during pregnancy induces neural and metabolic pathways in the fetus, predisposing the child, and even the future grandchild to obesity, before they have even taken a mouthful of food.

Research suggests that individuals are more receptive to, and more likely to act on, health messages that relate to areas of health where the individual perceives a personal risk. For example, someone who has recently had a heart attack and who is keen to ensure a reduction in serum cholesterol concentrations will respond to health messages – government sponsored or commercial advertising – that promise to produce such a reduction. Clearly, in such circumstances, the message is more likely to be acted upon even when, as may be the case for commercial companies, claims for outcomes cannot be guaranteed.[2]

Sadly government messages on nutrition may compete and conflict with commercial messages, and this only serves to increase the level of complexity and confusion, making it difficult or impossible for the public to know what strategy to adopt. In such situations ambivalence takes priority and change is avoided. This can be a particular problem for those more vulnerable members of society who have insufficient good information on which to make healthy choices.

Added to this is the fact that the general public are often suspicious of government-sponsored messages. Where government messages conflict with 'common sense', there is a high likelihood that the message will be ignored. Since government food messages, in the interests of scientific rigour, can become complex and difficult for the individual to decipher, let alone put into action, it is understandable that many fail to make healthy choices about their food.

Commercial organisations, when promoting foods, are less discerning about scientific rigour and more interested in the success of their product, irrespective of the health impact on the public. The Mars company, for example, were involved in a protracted legal battle with a primary health-care organisation, who were concerned about Mars' slogan, 'A Mars a day helps you work, rest and play'. The healthcare organisation felt that this was inappropriate and unproven and only served to encourage the public, particularly the more vulnerable, to consume more Mars bars than they should. Mars essentially won the case in that the judge ruled that, in small amounts, there was little evidence to suggest that Mars bars were damaging to health. An average member of the public would find this mixed message confusing and it may only serve to endorse a poor diet.[3]

Health messages concerning food may be difficult enough to communicate but health messages about food consumption and the maintenance of an ideal body weight become even more complex because a weight-reduction diet can be different from a healthy diet. Although both can, and ideally should, be the same, the public often find difficulty understanding the difference where it matters. For example, when asked, an average member of the public will identify brown bread as a healthier option than white bread; this message was successful communicated years ago. This answer will be based on the colour of the bread with little consideration of fibre content which, if absent, adds no health advantage.[4] Because the public believe that white bread is less healthy than brown there is an erroneous assumption, an incorrect causal link, that a slice of brown bread contains fewer calories than a slice of white bread. Similarly, 'low fat spreads' are only lower in calories compared with butter or margarine but spreads are still relatively calorie-dense and thus, when eaten in large amounts, will contribute to weight gain. A certain food may receive a green traffic light code on the label, but eating two 'greens' may make a 'red', which seems entirely illogical and counter-intuitive.

Such contradictions are common across the full food spectrum and it is increasingly clear that the public require constant reassurance and good-quality information on specific health aspects of the foods they eat. For pharmacists and other primary care professionals, good information on vitamin and mineral supplements is essential, as there exists a huge amount of misinformation and even unrealistic claims about these products.

Starvation diets

When attempting to lose weight, a strategy often adopted is to keep to the same diet but to eat less. This will be successful and can be sustained where

600 kcal are removed from the daily energy intake for a period of 6 months or more, coupled with an increase in daily exercise. Often, however, the individual retains the less healthy aspect of the diet, since he or she prefers these foods, and attempts to cut out more than the recommended 600 kcal, a strategy that is unsustainable in the long term.[5]

The key to success for a weight-reduction diet is to eat the ideal number of calories from the recommended food groups (see below). In this way the diet will be both healthy and weight reducing. All foods are composed mainly of carbohydrates, proteins or fats and it is the amounts of each of these contained within the food that determines the impact of the food on health. However, for weight reduction in obese individuals, more controversial and drastic methods may be appropriate.

For those people intending to lose weight on a simple hypocaloric diet, it is important to remember that 500–600 kcal are subtracted from their energy requirements, based on their age, gender, weight and level of activity, not on their current energy intake.

A person's energy requirements can be calculated using the modified Harris Benedict equation, in which basal metabolic rate (BMR) is multiplied by an activity factor (see Chapter 2, p. 36 for the BMR calculation). This gives the daily number of calories a person requires, and from which 500–600 kcal can then be subtracted.[6]

Food energy

About two-thirds of the energy the body uses goes into homeostasis, that is, keeping the body temperature constant, repairing tissues, maintaining heart and lung function and ensuring a proper chemical balance in the blood. Without considering physical activity, most adults need between 1300 kcal and 1800 kcal daily just to stay alive. For our normal daily activities, we need a further 500–1000 kcal. Of course our daily needs will depend on what activities we take part in during the day, our current body weight and for how long we do the activity.

Food types will differ in the energy per gram that they provide (table 10.1).

Table 10.1 Energy yield by food type	
Food	**Energy (kcals/gram)**
Fat	9
Protein	4
Carbohydrate	4
Alcohol	7

Carbohydrates

Breads and cereals are our main source of carbohydrates in the average diet and since they are also the least expensive, are relied on by most of the world's population to meet much of its daily energy requirement. Plants contain about 15% carbohydrate and are the main source.

Fruit and vegetables

In common with breads and cereals, fruit and vegetables are a good source of carbohydrates. The World Health Organization (WHO) suggests that 2.7 million lives could be saved each year if more fruit and vegetables were eaten.[7] Up to one-third of cancers are caused by dietary excursions and it is estimated that fruit and vegetable intake is only secondary to stopping smoking in reducing this cancer risk. The role of antioxidant vitamins in removing free radicals has been controversial but there is some evidence to support their role in reducing free-radical damage to cellular DNA. In addition, increased consumption of fruit and vegetables has been shown to reduce significantly the risk of coronary heart disease, cancer, obesity, raised blood pressure and there is even some evidence to suggest that there may be a reduced risk of Alzheimer's disease.

Both the WHO and the NHS advise eating a minimum of five 80-g portions of fruit or vegetables every day.[8] The government's National Diet and Nutrition Survey (2007)[9] showed that only 13% of men and 15% of women say that they comply with this target; the average is just 2.7 portions for men and 2.9 portions for women. Twenty-one per cent of men and 15% of women said they ate no fruit or vegetables at all. Even more shocking were the figures for men aged 19–24: none claimed to eat five portions, the average is 1.3 portions and 45% admitted to eating no fruit or vegetables at all.

Five portions is the minimum requirement – six, seven or eight or more would be better for the whole population. An easy way to measure a portion is if it fits into the hand. One portion is, for example:

- 1 apple
- 10 blackberries,
- 3 heaped tablespoons of cooked kidney beans.

It is important to vary the fruit and vegetables eaten and for this purpose the 'rainbow rule' was devised, which states that an individual should include red and orange vegetables and yellow, green and blue fruits as the range of antioxidants corresponds to their colour. In addition, a ratio of four portions of vegetables to three portions of fruit should be consumed daily. It should also be remembered that canned and frozen vegetables are an equally good substitute for fresh fruit and vegetables out of season, when they are more expensive.

For those individuals who prefer to sweeten their cereal, they should be encouraged do so with fruit rather than sugar. An ideal recommendation is to have two fruit snacks during the day and a lunch and dinner that has plenty of vegetables on the plate.

Vegetables lose water-soluble vitamins when boiled for a long periods but when eaten crunchy, the vitamin loss is reduced.

Potatoes are a starchy, carbohydrate food in the same category as bread and cereals and it is important that people appreciate that potatoes should not contribute to the daily fruit and vegetable intake. There is no evidence to suggest that organically grown vegetables are higher in nutrient content than non-organic foods and this must be balanced against the fact that organically grown vegetable are generally more expensive. Pure fruit juice and 'smoothies' (fruit put through a blender sometimes combined with yogurt) can count as a single daily portion but not more than one. When fruit is juiced through a blender, some of the nutritious plant chemicals and fibre in the cell walls are lost. There are also more higher natural sugars in juiced fruit which, when consumed in large quantities, can cause dental caries. Dried fruits are high in sugars and, although they have cardiometabolic benefits, their intake needs to be monitored.[10]

Protein foods

Meat is a main source of protein and, although associated with fat, the fat content of meat has dramatically reduced in lean meat over recent years. Dairy products can be a good source of protein but again there is an element of fat. Beans, nuts and cereal grains are also a good protein source and associated fats are generally lower and seldom saturated. In developed nations, a higher proportion of protein in the diet comes from meat and dairy products, where it is combined with fat. This contrasts with less-developed nations, where the main source of protein is plants.

Dairy products, fats and added sugars

Milk, cream and cheese provide nearly 60% of dietary calcium. Cooking oil, lard, butter, margarine, *ghee* (popular in Indian cooking) and shortening are almost pure fat. Foods that contain a large amount of fat include dairy products, chocolate, cakes, pies, cookies, nuts and, surprisingly, some fruits such as coconut and avocado. Coconut oil is solid at room temperature, demonstrating its properties as a saturated fat, with all the associated health disadvantages.[11]

Red–green–amber food labelling

An energy-based food-exchange system has been developed that divides foods into five groups[12]:

- *Carbohydrates* – including bread, pasta and potatoes. They are high in starch and provide energy through the breakdown of starch into sugars.
- *Fruit and vegetables* – rich in vitamins and minerals. A target should be to eat at least five, but preferably as many portions of fruit and vegetables as possible each day. One portion counts as one glass of fruit juice (which counts once only), a large piece of fruit such as an apple or banana, or three heaped tablespoons of vegetables.
- *Protein* – good sources include meat, fish, eggs, beans and nuts. Proteins help to build and repair the body and should make up one-fifth of the diet.
- *Dairy* – cheese, milk and yoghurt are all dairy foods and are rich in calcium, important for strong bones and teeth.
- *Fats and added sugar* – including butter, chocolate, crisps and cakes. These foods typically contain a lot of fat and added sugar. Fats are divided into two groups – saturated and unsaturated. Saturated fat is found in cream, margarine and fried foods – and this type of fat can contribute to coronary heart disease and cancer. Unsaturated fat is found in vegetable oils and oily fish. Eating a small amount of these fats can help to keep the immune system healthy. Added sugars should be eaten sparingly because they contribute to health problems and are high in calories.

The foods in each group are colour coded according to nutrient density: green for 'go', yellow for 'eat with care', and red for 'stop'. 'Green' foods are foods containing fewer than 20 kcal per serving, 'yellow' foods are the staple of the diet and provide most of the basic nutrition, and 'red' foods are those foods high in fat and simple carbohydrates. All sweets and sugared beverages are classified as 'red' foods. Families instructed to count calories should not have more than four 'red' foods a week.

Standard UK population recommendations on 'healthy eating' are based on the recommendations of the Committee on the Medical Aspects of Food Policy and subsequently the Scientific Advisory Committee on Nutrition.[13] The recommendations are summarised in table 10.2.

These recommendations do not apply to children under 2 years of age. Between 2 and 5 years of age, a flexible approach to the timing and extent of dietary change should be taken. By the age of 5 years, children should be consuming a diet consistent with the recommendations for adults.

Table 10.2 Standard population dietary recommendations	
Nutrient/food	**Recommendation**
Total fat	Reduce to no more than 35% food energy
Saturated fat	Reduce to no more than 11% food energy
Total carbohydrate	Increase to more than 50% food energy
Sugars (added)	Reduce to no more than 11% food energy
Dietary fibre	Increase non-starch polysaccharides to 18 g/day
Salt	Reduce to no more than 6 g/day*
Fruit and vegetables	Increase to at least five portions of a variety of fruit and vegetables per day

*The maximum amount of salt recommended for children is less than that for adults.

This advice is reflected in the 'eatwell plate'[14] (figure 10.1), but should be regarded as a means of maintaining health rather than reducing obesity. The Food Standards Agency[14] summarises the advice as:

- Base your meals on starchy foods.
- Eat lots of fruit and vegetables.
- Eat fish – including a portion of oily fish each week.
- Minimise saturated fat and sugar.
- Try to eat less salt – no more than a maximum of 6 g a day for adults.

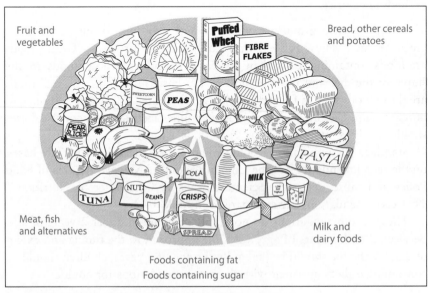

Figure 10.1 The eatwell plate. From Food Standards Agency.[14]

- Get active and try to be a healthy weight.
- Drink plenty of water.
- Don't skip breakfast.
- And remember to enjoy your food!

With regard to the prevention of obesity, WHO says that 'there is convincing evidence that a high intake of energy dense foods promotes weight gain' and that 'the majority of studies show that a high intake of NSP (dietary fibre) promotes weight loss'.[8] This report confirms that energy-dense foods tend to be high in fat (e.g. butter, oils, fried foods), sugars or starch, while energy-dilute foods have a high fibre and water content (e.g. fruit and vegetables, whole grain cereals). The report concluded that there was 'probable' evidence that increased consumption of sweetened drinks and large portion sizes increases the risk of weight gain and obesity. Sugar-based drinks are a particular problem in that they are energy-dense yet they fail to affect satiety triggers that would reduce food intake. In this way a large serving of a sugar-based drink could amount to 400 kcal, yet when consumed it would not trigger satiety so eating can continue.

Dietary advice

A key component in losing weight and maintaining a healthy level is to ensure that dietary advice is tailored for the individual. The following is the National Institute for Health and Clinical Excellence (NICE) guidance on a weight reduction diet.[16] The diet should take account of food preferences and allow for a flexible approach in reducing energy intake. When the diet is restrictive, the individual will simply not stick with it and when the diet is nutritionally unbalanced, the diet can be harmful.

Low-carbohydrate diets are being increasingly recommended for the management of obesity and insulin resistance[17], and have been shown to be superior to other regimes at 6 months, and at least as good after one year. Other risk factors such as blood pressure and lipid profile also improve significantly. It is important to combine low carbohydrate with low fat, rather than deliberately increasing fat consumption as some commercial initiatives have done, and also to ensure a healthy level of fruit and vegetable intake.

People should be encouraged to improve their diet, even if they do not lose weight, because there can be other health benefits. The main requirement of a dietary approach to weight loss is that total energy intake should be less than energy expenditure. Diets that have a 600 kcal per day deficit compared with the person's energy requirement or diets that reduce energy by lowering the fat content (low-fat diets), in combination with expert support and intensive follow up, are recommended for sustainable weight loss.

Low-energy diets (1000–1600 kcal per day) may also be considered, but are less likely to be nutritionally complete, although commercial low- and very-low-energy diets include sufficient nutritional supplementation to ensure that no nutrients are lacking. Very-low-energy diets (fewer than 1000 kcal per day), may be used for a maximum of 12 weeks continuously, or intermittently with a low-energy diet (for example for 2–4 days a week) by people who are obese and have reached a plateau in weight loss.[15] Any diet of fewer than 600 kcal per day should be used only under clinical supervision. Commercial low- and very-low-energy diet programmes include psychological input in order that long-term weight loss is more likely to be maintained.

Meal replacement regimes, which replace one or two meals per day with a low-energy drink or snack, are backed by robust long-term evidence[18] and may be useful interventions. In the longer term, people should move towards eating a balanced diet, consistent with other healthy eating advice.

Children

A dietary approach alone is not recommended. It is essential that any dietary recommendations are part of a multi-component intervention. Any dietary changes should be age-appropriate and consistent with healthy eating advice.

For overweight and obese children and adolescents, total energy intake should be below their energy expenditure. Changes should be sustainable.

Pregnancy and breastfeeding

Healthy nutrition is a lifelong matter and during the course of our lives, our nutritional requirements change and, if we wish to remain healthy, so too should our diets. 'Epigenetics' describes how the environment can permanently alter our gene expression, for example, even in the uterus the mother's diet will have a permanent impact on the developing fetus. Neural and metabolic pathways are forged *in utero*, which influence future generations of offspring; there is clear evidence that a mother's diet during pregnancy can influence the child's diet and predisposition to obesity later on. For example, children of a group of mothers who eat a diet that contained a high level of vegetables during pregnancy were more likely to include vegetables in their diets later in life.

Breastfed babies are less likely to be overweight and are less likely to become fat children and subsequently fat babies are more likely to grow into overweight and obese adults. There are significant other advantages from breastfeeding, including an enhanced immune system – antibodies are transferred in breast milk, particularly in colostrum, the rich, thick, yellowish milk produced before mature milk comes in. It is thought to protect against infection and asthma and childhood eczema. Furthermore a breastfeeding mother is more likely to regain her pre-pregnancy weight than mothers who bottle feed.

The presence of the 'C' version of the gene FADS2, found in 90% of children, boosts a breastfed baby's IQ by seven points. This gene is responsible for the metabolism of fatty acids in the diet and breast milk is a rich source of fatty acids. It is felt that in this way certain aspects of brain development are enhanced in breastfed babies.[19]

In England in 2005, 77% of babies were breastfed at birth but this falls to 55% at 1 week and more than 33% of mothers stop within the first 6 weeks. Both prevalence and duration of breastfeeding in the UK are the lowest in Europe. There is a social gradient present, with 90% of mothers in professional groups initiating breastfeeding, whereas in manual classes only 60% start.[20]

A study presented in 2007 to the American Heart Association[21] has shown that breastfeeding is linked with lower weight and higher high-density lipoprotein cholesterol in adulthood as well as a lower risk of developing heart disease.

To tackle our current obesity problem successfully, there needs to be a renewed commitment to increasing the number of mothers who breastfeed their babies and to supporting them to do this for longer.

Pharmacy HealthLink

The PharmacyHealthLink (http://www.pharmacyhealthlink.org.uk/) provides nutritional guidance for pharmacists. The most important aspects of a healthy diet are summarised as:

- choosing foods in the right proportions from the five main food groups
- eating a varied diet to obtain essential vitamins and minerals
- limiting the consumption of other foodstuffs in addition to main meals – especially those that are high in energy, have little nutritional benefit and can cause health problems in the longer term, e.g. salt and alcohol.

The diet should provide sufficient nutrients and maintain health. For those who are overweight or obese, low-fat and reduced-sugar foods will accelerate weight loss. People should be encouraged to eat five portions of fruit and vegetables per day; these can be raw, cooked, canned, frozen or dried and one portion may be substituted with a glass of fruit juice if preferred. The crude but useful description of one portion is a handful; therefore a normal-sized apple orange or pear will be one portion (box 10.1).

> *Box 10.1* *Principles of good dietary management*
> - Avoid or correct obesity by reducing energy intake.
> - Increase percentage of energy from high-fibre carbohydrates so that carbohydrate intake accounts for at least 50% of energy intake.
> - Reduce fats to 30% of total energy; saturated fats should account for 10% of total energy.
> - Restrict maximum protein content of food to 20% of energy intake.
> - Distribute food intake easily throughout the day, and reasonably consistently from day to day.

Vitamins and minerals

Eating a balanced, but varied, diet should give most people the range of vitamins and minerals that they need. Vitamins are compounds essential in small amounts to maintain normal health and development. Our bodies are a well-organised factory system: the 'workers' breaking down food and building up new tissue are the body's enzymes. As with all good workers, enzymes need tools to perform their task efficiently. Vitamins, also called co-enzymes, provide these tools and, since they are very efficient tools, they are only required in small amounts.

The following section is an updated version of a previously published paper.[22]

As a general rule, the body is unable to manufacture vitamins and therefore they must be ingested in the diet. Shortage of a vitamin hampers the work of its associated enzyme, resulting in a number of body components not being produced or not being broken down. In the short term, this may not be a problem and a temporary lack of a vitamin may only give rise to minor symptoms which disappear with a return to a good diet. However when the deficiency lasts for a longer time, the condition become a deficiency disease, for example, scurvy caused by a lack of vitamin C, rickets by a lack of vitamin D, beriberi by a lack of vitamin B and night-blindness caused by a lack of vitamin A.

Some minerals act as co-enzymes in the same way as vitamins do; other minerals are components of larger body molecules, such as iron in haemo-globin, and are therefore vital for good health.

Who needs supplements?

Dietary supplement is the general term given to products designed to be adjuncts to the diet but these substances are usually present in the diet anyway, so supplementation is generally unnecessary. Certain categories of people may benefit from supplements, however. These include children up to the age of 12 years, pregnant women, people recovering from illness and the elderly. Generally a multivitamin preparation with minerals would be sufficient – these contain small but sufficient amounts of all important vitamins and minerals.

Elderly people tend to eat less since they have a reduced appetite, many have dentures which makes chewing difficult, and many neglect themselves, living on a limited diet. They may be physically incapable of shopping or cooking or cannot afford to buy fresh food. For these reasons, vitamin supplements are a good idea for many elderly people, who are particularly prone to shortage of vitamin C.

Those on very-low-energy diets and vegetarians might also benefit from multivitamin supplementation.

Vitamin fact file

Vitamins are divided into 'fat-soluble' and 'water-soluble'. Vitamins A, D, E and K are the main fat-soluble vitamins and they tend to accumulate in the body, especially in the liver, which acts as a store in case of shortage. Fat-soluble vitamins can be toxic in high doses and it is important that the public are aware of the recommended daily dose. The other vitamins are water-soluble and as a result more easily lost from the body. They are not stored effectively and therefore deficiencies can occur. Some of the water-soluble vitamins – for example, vitamin C – appear to be well tolerated in very high doses but others can cause side-effects at high concentrations – for example, vitamin B_6 causes nerve damage at high doses.

Vitamin A

Vitamin A (retinol and carotene) helps to improve the body's resistance to disease and helps skin condition. It is essential for the growth of teeth and bone and for the replacement of the surface layers of skin, both externally and internally. Internal surfaces include the lining of the respiratory passages, the mucous lining of the gut and the tracts of the urinary and genital organs. The cells on these surfaces need to be constantly replaced and vitamin A has a major role to play in this.

Vitamin A is also found in the eye as a precursor of rhodopsin, which allows sight in conditions of low light. Deficiency of vitamin A will lead to night blindness.

The recommended daily amount of vitamin A for health is 0.75 mg and since it can be stored in the liver, most people have sufficient supplies. An excessive intake of vitamin A can be dangerous, causing sickness, dizziness and dermatitis. Indeed toxic levels can be achieved in those using high-dose supplements. High doses are also related to birth defects and those wishing to or at risk of becoming pregnant should be advised not to use supplements.

Vitamin A is available in liver, butter, carrots, potatoes and leafy green vegetables. Retinol is found in animal products while carotene, which is converted to vitamin A in the body, is found in fruit and vegetables.

Vitamin B

Vitamin B is a complex of vitamins: B_1, B_2, niacin, B_5, B_6, folic acid, B_{12} and biotin, with an interdependency on each other so that a deficiency in one can affect the activity of others.

Vitamin B_1 (thiamine) is primarily involved in the production of energy in the body and the daily requirement is determined by the calories that we consume in our diet. A deficiency interferes with metabolism of glucose to pyruvate and can lead to an increase in blood pressure and oedema. This latter symptom is the starting point for beriberi, the vitamin B_1 deficiency disease, producing neuropathy and myopathy. Rare in the UK, these symptoms are seen in a milder form in alcoholic patients, who are prone to deficiencies in vitamin B.

The richest sources of vitamin B_1 are seeds, nuts, peas, beans, cereals and yeast. Fish and meat, especially pork, are all good sources. Vitamin B_1 0.4 mg is needed for every 1000 kcal consumed in the diet, giving a recommended daily requirement of 1.0–1.2 mg daily. Vitamin B_1 is easily destroyed in the cooking of food.

Vitamin B_2 (riboflavin) plays an important part in oxygen utilisation. Deficiencies are linked to soreness of mouth and tongue. The recommended daily amount for health is 1.2 mg a day for adults. Vitamin B_2 is found in cereals but is more plentiful in dairy products and meat. Kidney, fish, yeast extract (Marmite) and nuts are particularly rich sources.

Niacin (nicotinic acid) is a B vitamin not assigned a number. It protects against pellagra, a skin disease that affects communities dependent on maize as a main source of food. Symptoms include severe dermatitis and reddening of the skin. Niacin is found in meat, fish, whole cereal and yeast. A good supply can be obtained from liver, kidney, beans, peas, nuts, dried fruits and fresh fruits and vegetables. Niacin is used in high dose (3 g per day) and under medical supervision for lowering cholesterol.

Vitamin B_6 (pyridoxine) is important in the building of protein structures from amino acids and in the development of neurotransmitter substances. Deficiency produces a form of anaemia caused by a lack of haemoglobin.

Good sources of vitamin B$_6$ include yeast, liver, wholegrains, peanuts and bananas. The recommended daily intake is 1–2 mg.

Vitamin B$_{12}$ (cyanocobalamin) and folate are necessary for blood cell and nerve tissues development and deficiencies are linked with megaloblastic anaemia. When folate supplements are given, it speeds up red blood cell formation to such an extent that vitamin B$_{12}$ is withdrawn from nervous tissue, being redirected to red blood cell formation and, as a result, can lead to nerve damage.

Vitamin B$_{12}$ is only found in animal tissue. This theoretically causes a problem for strict vegetarians such as vegans, as they have no obvious source of this vitamin. Interestingly, such individuals rarely suffer from vitamin B$_{12}$ deficiency and it has been suggested that accidental ingestion of insects provide sufficient vitamin B$_{12}$ to avoid deficiency.

Biotin is widely distributed among all types of food so again it is unlikely that on a normal diet anyone would go short. However, avidin, a substance found in raw egg white (it is denatured by cooking), combines with biotin and stops it being absorbed. This type of deficiency causes severe eczema in those eccentric people who live on a diet of raw eggs and whisky!

Vitamin C

Vitamin C (ascorbic acid) is needed in the production of collagen, a material that literally 'cements' the body together. Scurvy is the disease that results from a deficiency. As a result, the skin can no longer act as a barrier against infection. The walls of small blood vessels become weak and break down causing bruising and help the spread of the infection. Bleeding gums are a common feature and poor wound healing makes minor cuts and bruises a problem. Additionally, vitamin C works closely in association with white blood cells in the elimination of bacteria. It is also involved in the formation of bone where it assists in the deposition of minerals to form healthy bones.

Potatoes, green vegetables, fresh fruit, meat and milk are all good sources of vitamin C and a balanced diet containing these foods should easily provide the 30 mg daily requirement we each need.

Vitamin D

Vitamin D (dihyroxycholecalciferol) is unusual in that it is not an essential requirement in the diet, as the skin using sunlight can make this vitamin. The main role for vitamin D is to increase absorption of calcium from the gut. A deficiency in vitamin D will cause rickets because of its role in bone metabolism and this can occur where sunlight levels are low and vitamin D levels in the diet are below the required level.

Fish oils, dairy products, liver and kidney are rich sources of vitamin D. Since it is a fat-soluble vitamin, it is stored in the liver and supplied during times of shortage. The vitamin is toxic in high concentration and can cause symptoms of sickness, dizziness and diarrhoea. Breastfeeding women in particular must be cautioned about not exceeding the recommended daily intake of fish oil supplements, as vitamin D may affect the growing baby.

Vitamin E

Vitamin E (α-tocopherol) is another fat-soluble vitamin that is stored in the liver and is seldom associated with deficiency. It has a role as the precursor of antioxidants and there is speculation that it might act against the development of cancers, although evidence is not very strong. Vitamin E is found in eggs, butter, vegetable oils, green leafy vegetables and cereals.

Vitamin K

Vitamin K is involved with normal blood clotting. Fortunately vitamin K is normally in plentiful supply as gut bacteria manufacture it and, as a result, deficiency is rare. Vitamin K is found in green-leafed vegetables such as broccoli, kale and spinach.

Other foodstuffs

It is important to encourage people to think about other foodstuffs that they eat on a regular basis, for example, alcohol, soft drinks and salt are commonly consumed in addition to meals and have specific health effects.

Salt

A reduction in the average intake of the overall population from 9 g to 6 g per day would result in an estimated reduced incidence of coronary heart disease by 6%, stroke by 15% and hypertension by 17%.[23] As most salt in the diet (around 75%) is obtained from processed food, the easiest ways to cut down on salt are choosing foods with reduced salt content (usually listed as 'sodium' in the food label) and by not adding salt to cooking or at the table. The recommended daily levels of salt are 6 g for an adult. The daily recommended maximum for children depends on their age.

- 1 to 3 years: 2 g (0.8 g sodium)
- 4 to 6 years: 3 g (1.2 g sodium)
- 7 to 10 years: 5 g (2 g sodium)
- 11 and over: 6 g (2.5 g sodium)

Alcohol

The Department of Health advises that men should not drink more than 3–4 units of alcohol per day, and women should drink no more than 2–3 units of alcohol per day. This recommendation has changed from previous recommendations of 28 units of alcohol per week for men and 21 units of alcohol per week for women. In the new recommendations, the daily benchmark applies whether individuals drink every day, once or twice a week, or only occasionally.

Alcohol can provide a very high number of calories depending on what people drink and how much. Lager, beer and stout have the highest energy content per drink and can range from 170 to 400 kcal per pint. Therefore it is possible to exceed the maximum daily energy intake (2000 kcal a day for women and 2500 kcal a day for men) with alcohol alone.

A unit of alcohol is a half a pint of standard strength (3–5% ABV) beer, lager or cider or a pub measure of spirit (not in Northern Ireland). A glass of wine is about 2 units and a glass of 'alcopops' is about 1.5 units.

Soft drinks

Fizzy drinks, squashes, 'sports' and 'high juice' drinks all count as soft drinks. They are typically high in sugar and therefore calories and have very little nutritional content in contrast to 100% fruit juice and smoothies. They also tend to be acidic, which can cause tooth decay and enamel erosion if consumed regularly between meals. Healthier alternatives are water, milk and fruit juices (ideally consumed with a meal).

The satiety value of sugary soft drinks is less than for the equivalent for solid forms.

Tips for a healthy diet

- Take time to enjoy your food – but aim to stay a 'healthy weight'.
- Eat a variety of foodstuffs but choose them mainly from the healthy food groups.
- Avoid food and drinks with a high fat or sugar content.
- Choose foods that are rich in starch and fibre as these will fill you up more easily than fatty or sugary foods.
- Eat at least one portion of fruit and vegetables a day, but aim for five.

Easy ways to eat more fruit and vegetables:

- Choose fresh fruit for desserts or instead of crisps and chocolate.
- Have a glass of fruit juice instead of tea, coffee or fizzy drinks.
- Eat salad at least once a day.

- Put fresh or frozen vegetables into soups, pasta or noodles.
- Top pizzas with extra vegetables such as peppers, mushrooms and tomatoes.
- Mix fruit into yoghurts.

What is a portion of fruit or vegetables?

- 1 apple, pear, orange, banana or other similar sized fruit
- 2 plums or similar sized fruit
- half a grapefruit or avocado
- 1 slice of large fruit such as melon or pineapple
- 3 tablespoons of vegetables (raw, cooked, frozen or canned)
- 3 tablespoons of beans and pulses (however much you eat, beans and pulses count for just one portion per day)
- 3 tablespoons of fruit salad (fresh or canned in fruit juice) or stewed fruit
- 1 tablespoon of dried fruit such as raisins or 3 whole apricots
- A handful of grapes, cherries or berries
- A cereal bowl of mixed salad
- A glass (150 mL) of fruit juice (however much you drink, fruit juice counts as just one portion a day).

References

1. Haslam D. *Obesity: your questions answered*. Oxford: Radcliffe Medical Press, 2006.
2. Sherman M *et al*. Approach/avoidance motivation, message framing and health behaviour. *Motiv Emot* 2006; 30: 165–169.
3. Krebs J. Food advertising and health, 2007. http://www.epublichealth.org.uk.
4. Renfrew M *et al*. *The Effectiveness of Public Health Interventions*. London: NICE, 2005.
5. National Institute for Health and Clinical Excellence. Guidance on diet. London: NICE.
6. Douglas C *et al*. Ability of the Harris-Benedict formula to predict energy requirements differs with weight history and ethnicity. *Nutr Res* 2000; 27: 194–199.
7. World Health Organization/Food & Agricultural Organization. *Diet, Nutrition and the Prevention of Chronic Diseases*. WHO Technical Report Series 916. Geneva: WHO/FAO, 2003.
8. World Health Organization. *Obesity: preventing and managing the global epidemic*. WHO Technical Report Series 894, I-253. Geneva: WHO, 2003.
9. Food Standards Agency. *National Diet and Nutrition Survey (Adult)*. London: The Stationary Office, 2007.
10. Bender A. *Introduction to Nutrition and Metabolism*, 2nd edn. London: Taylor & Francis Ltd, 1997.
11. Health Education Authority. *Scientific Basis of Nutrition Education*. Melksham: Cromwell Press, 1996.
12. Epstein L *et al*. Treatment of pediatric obesity. *Pediatrics* 1998; 101(Suppl): 554–570.
13. Aggett P. *et al*. Recommended Dietary Allowances (RDAs), Recommended Dietary Intakes (RDIs), Recommended Nutrient Intakes (RNIs) and Population Reference Intakes (PRIs) are not 'Recommended Intakes'. *J Pediatr Gastroenterol Nutr* 1997; 25: 236–241.
14. Food Standards Agency. The eatwell plate. http://www.eatwell.gov.uk (accessed 10 Jul 2009).

15. National Institute for Health and Clinical Excellence. Obesity: the prevention, identification, assessment and management of overweight and obesity in adults and children. *Clinical Guidance* 2006; 43.

16. National Audit Office. *Tackling Obesity in England.* London: The Stationery Office, 2001.

17. Parke S *et al.* Some taste molecules and their solution properties. *Chem Senses* 1999; 24: 271–279.

18. Koplman P *et al.* eds. *Clinical Obesity in Adults and Children,* 2nd edn. Oxford: Blackwell, 2007.

19. Xie L, Innis S. Genetic variants of the FADS1 FADS2 gene cluster are associated with altered (n-6) and (n-3) essential fatty acids in plasma and erythrocyte phospholipids in women during pregnancy and in breast milk during lactation. *J Nutr* 2008; 138: 2222–2228.

20. American Academy of Pediatrics. Breastfeeding and the use of human milk. Policy statement. *Pediatrics* 2005; 115: 496–506.

21. Tennant R *et al.* Barriers to breastfeeding. *Community Practitioner* 2006; 79: 152–156.

22. Maguire T. Vitamins and minerals. *Pharm J* 1996; 256.

23. Department of Health. *Choosing Health: making healthier choices easier.* London: Department of Health, 2004.

11

Pharmacological interventions

Whereas debate may continue on whether obesity is a disease, a syndrome or a natural response to an abnormal environment, there remains little disagreement on the causal link between obesity and morbidity and mortality. In simple terms, as an individual amasses body fat, the risk of disease increases. Logically therefore, as with other conditions such as raised blood pressure, which is also associated with an increased disease risk, effective pharmacological intervention should be provided when such an intervention substantially reduces that disease risk. Certainly for raised blood pressure, the case for pharmacological intervention was proven long ago. Lifestyle change can reduce blood pressure but the relevant intervention data are less impressive than those which support pharmacological treatment, and certainly compliance is poorer, so pharmacological intervention is more likely to be successful in reducing disease risk.

For obesity, the question whether pharmacological or lifestyle intervention is superior has been answered in that lifestyle intervention – better diet and increased activity – have been proved effective in reducing morbidity and mortality. We are only now beginning to amass data that support the reduced disease risk induced by licensed pharmacotherapy, yet this is still only to a limited extent. The greater this evidence becomes over time, the more widespread the use of pharmacological interventions will become, yet it is likely that this use will always be in conjunction with lifestyle changes. For this reason, practitioners continue to place a priority on lifestyle modification, which is key to sustainable weight reduction, with pharmacotherapy being reserved for those who cannot significantly reduce disease risk by lifestyle change alone.

Whereas the risks associated with obesity increase alongside weight gain in a linear fashion, the risk reduction with weight loss, with or without medication, is much more dramatic in scale than the actual degree of weight lost. A loss of 10% of body weight equates to a loss of 3% of visceral fat, which is accompanied by a dramatic reduction in disease risk. Yet it must be remembered, particularly with regard to older agents now no longer used, that even where a drug is capable of affecting a 5% or 10% weight loss, this does not necessarily mean that this weight loss reduces an individual's disease risk by the same percentage. For example, a side-effect of the drug could also increase a patient's cardiovascular risk to the extent that it offsets any health benefit and therefore, in such a case, use of the medicine could not be justified. Indeed it is for this very reason that many drugs effective in reducing weight are no longer recommended for use in the management of obesity.[1] Even those that are currently licensed for this indication remain under surveillance.

Who should use pharmacotherapy?

It is appreciated that many obese people are unable to achieve and sustain weight loss through lifestyle modification alone. Individuals with insulin resistance, for instance, have been shown to lose weight only half as successfully as others, by whichever means is attempted. The National Institute for Health and Clinical Excellence (NICE) advises that drug therapy should be considered for patients who have not reached their target weight loss, or have reached a plateau with dietary, activity and behavioural change alone.[2] This endorsement of pharmacological intervention, albeit with some reservations, has fuelled an increase in prescriptions for the two drugs currently available; orlistat (Xenical), and sibutramine (Reductil). Rimonabant (Acomplia) had its marketing authorisation suspended in October 2008 but is considered in this chapter since that licence may yet be reinstated because of the highly significant benefits it induces and extremely positive NICE verdict, despite the fact that all Phase III trials have, at the time of writing, been terminated. These three medicines have been introduced relatively recently but follow a long list of pharmacological agents that were indicated and used for the management of obesity and which were successful to a degree but withdrawn because of side-effects.

Some of the most toxic substances known have historically been used to induce weight reduction, including mercury, arsenic, strychnine and dinitrophenol. Perhaps the most notorious of the anti-obesity medicines were the amphetamines (e.g. Dexamyl, Eskatrol, Dexedrine, Didrex)[1] some of which, to compound the felony, were combined with barbiturates (Ambar) in order to minimise side-effects. The noradrenergic appetite suppressants, phentermine and diethylpropion, are still widely used for weight loss in the US, although their use is limited because of adverse effects and they can only be used in the short term (a few weeks). Phentermine and diethylpropion are not prescribable on the National Health Service in the UK because the evidence base for their use in long-term obesity management is non-existent, despite being used for over 40 years. They are, however, still prescribed privately, usually at great expense to the patient and ensuring considerable profit for the practitioner, through a regulatory loophole. Interestingly, a brief ban on the drugs a few years ago was overturned on the basis that it was considered illegal to use the same evidence used to launch a drug, to subsequently ban it. Phentermine is commonly used in the US and elsewhere for rapid short-term loss but rapid and rebound weight gain associated with its use remains problematic. Many are willing to pay for and risk the use of these drugs because, for many individuals, obesity is a vanity issue rather than a health issue.

There also exists an extensive range of over-the-counter (OTC) remedies for weight loss and, although most of these may have few side-effects, it is likely that this is because they have little efficacy, the exception being Alli (orlistat 60 mg) which was launched as an OTC medicine across Europe in April 2009. OTC remedies are covered in detail in Chapter 14.

Drugs currently licensed for management of obesity – orlistat and sibutramine – are effective in reducing body weight and reducing risk parameters but neither as yet have specific outcomes data on, for instance, reduction of cardiovascular events. Yet, in the absence of complete data, it is a safe assumption that weight reduction using these agents is associated with a improvement in disease risk. Most studies involving these drugs had weight loss as a primary outcome but secondary outcomes such as changes in lipid profiles and serum glucose control suggest that there may indeed be benefits in reduced disease risk in addition to weight loss.

The most recent addition to the armoury of anti-obesity drugs is the partial-endocannabinoid receptor blocker, rimonabant, the evidence for which comes primarily from the Phase III Rimonabant In Obesity (RIO) trials. In the 2-year RIO–Europe Study[3], rimonabant 20 mg was shown to induce significantly greater improvements in waist circumference, high-density lipoprotein cholesterol, triglycerides and insulin resistance than placebo, associated with a reduced prevalence of metabolic syndrome incidence maintained up to at least 24 months. Other RIO studies showed a reduction in the percentage of individuals fulfilling the criteria for metabolic syndrome of around 57% on treatment with rimonabant compared with around 31% with placebo.

Data from the RIO diabetes trials indicate that rimonabant delivers a significant reduction in glycosylated haemoglobin HbA_{1c} of 0.7% reduction versus placebo, and that 43% of patients achieved an HbA_{1c} concentration of less than 6.5%. There was also a 15.4% increase in high-density lipoprotein from baseline along with a 9% decrease in triglycerides. The recently presented SERENADE trial studied the effects of rimonabant on drug-naive patients with diabetes, reporting significant reductions in HbA_{1c} from 8.5% by an average 1.9%.[4] These findings are particularly of interest to primary care, as the drug was shown to act upon a level of HbA_{1c} well outside the Quality and Outcomes Framework limits, often representing deteriorating disease, potentially bringing it down to well within General Medical Services specifications. Approximately 50% of the effect of rimonabant on risk markers is over and above that which would be anticipated by weight loss alone.

The most robust evidence for orlistat is a placebo-controlled trial in obese patients where, at 4 years, the weight loss caused by orlistat plus lifestyle changes was associated with a 37% lower cumulative incidence of diabetes, which is encouraging; however, this difference was only in a subgroup of patients with impaired glucose tolerance.[5] For rimonabant and sibutramine, the longest duration of fully published randomised controlled trials (RCTs) is currently only 2 years.

In recent years, there has been a marked increase in the prescribing of these medicines, with about one million prescription items for obesity dispensed in 2007, more than eight times the amount prescribed in 1999. Orlistat accounted for about 67% of prescriptions, sibutramine 24% and rimonabant 9%.

On average, the two currently licensed anti-obesity agents, orlistat and sibutramine, and rimonabant achieved weight reduction of less than 5 kg according to a meta-analysis.[6] Cardiovascular risk profiles differed across these agents. In particular it has been shown that, whereas cardiovascular risk factors including blood pressure were reduced in patients who lost weight using orlistat, a similar reduction was not found in patients whose weight loss was achieved using sibutramine. It is well established that sibutramine causes a rise in blood pressure and pulse rate in a small number of patients.

NICE guidance

It is illogical to use pharmacological agents for the management of obesity in the absence of behavioural modification. In the UK, NICE supports the use of orlistat (Xenical) and sibutramine (Reductil) in specific circumstances and has issued guidelines for their use in primary care.

NICE emphasises that drugs should be prescribed only as part of an overall plan for managing obesity.[2] This includes having arrangements in place to provide patients with information, support and counselling on additional diet, physical activity and behavioural strategies. Treatment should be reviewed regularly to monitor for effectiveness, adverse effects and adherence, and lifestyle advice should be reinforced at the same time.

NICE recommends that treatment with orlistat or sibutramine for longer than 3 months should be considered only if the person has lost at least 5% of their initial body weight since starting drug treatment. Orlistat may be continued for longer than a year, but only after discussing its risks and benefits with the patient. However, sibutramine treatment is not recommended beyond the licensed duration of 1 year.

Support should be given to patients who withdraw from treatment, as they may have low self-confidence, especially if they did not reach their target weight. People with type 2 diabetes may lose weight more slowly and so less strict goals may need to be agreed. It should be remembered that drug treatment can be used to help maintain weight loss as well as to help people to continue to lose weight. It is often the case that patients regain weight once anti-obesity drugs are stopped, in the same way that blood pressure will increase once a hypotensive agent is discontinued, or cholesterol following statin withdrawal.

Although drugs cannot replace exercise and adoption of a energy-deficient diet and should not be used alone, drug therapy is appropriate as long as it is done in accordance with current recommendations and with coordinated support for the patient. After 1 year of treatment, the weight loss induced above that achieved by diet and lifestyle management is 2.9 kg for orlistat, 4.2 kg for sibutramine and 4.7 kg for rimonabant.[6,7]

In clinical trials, patients taking drug therapy in addition to lifestyle changes (which include a hypocaloric diet) lose an average of approximately 3–5 kg more weight than with placebo in the first year. However in real life practice, rather than in a pharmaceutical trial environment, there is a wide spectrum of weight loss, or even gain, and the concept of 'average weight loss' on which the success of a drug trial is judged, is meaningless. The fact is that a non-responder will lose no weight, or possibly gain, then the obvious obverse consequence is that responders will lose far more weight than trials suggest. Assuming that non-responders are taken off the medication, then only those who are experiencing highly significant benefits will remain on treatment. When treatment is continued during the second year, drug treatment can help to maintain the initial weight loss seen, even if patients regain some weight and there is no good evidence that continued treatment with anti-obesity drugs over several years leads to additional weight loss beyond that seen in the first year.

Orlistat

Orlistat (Xenical 120-mg capsules) was first licensed in the UK in 1999. Its mechanism of action is inhibition of gastric, pancreatic and carboxylester lipases in the stomach lumen and the small intestine. The drug covalently binds to the lipase enzymes inhibiting their action. As a result, triglycerides in the diet cannot be enzymatically degraded into absorbable, free fatty acids and the amount of fat left unabsorbed is increased to 30% compared with around 4% in the absence of the drug. Owing to this local mechanism of action and subsequent negligible systemic absorption, orlistat does not accumulate in the body, even with long-term treatment. Orlistat improves some serum lipid values more than can be explained by weight reduction alone and may be particularly useful in obese patients with dyslipidaemia.

NICE guidance

NICE advises that orlistat can be used in patients aged between 18 and 75 years with a BMI of at least 30 kg/m², or 28 kg/m² in the presence of associated risk factors, such as type 2 diabetes, hypertension or hyperlipidaemia.

The prescribed dose is 120 mg three times daily with meals (dose should be omitted if a meal is missed or if there is no fat in the meal). Therapy should be continued for beyond 3 months only if the person has lost at least 5% of their initial body weight since starting drug treatment. The decision to use drug treatment for longer than 12 months (usually for weight maintenance) should be made after discussing potential benefits and limitations with the patient.

Clinical trials

A meta-analysis assessed 16 RCTs (n = 10 631) of orlistat.[7] At 1 year, patients in the orlistat group lost 2.9 kg more of their body weight compared with those on placebo. Also, compared with placebo, 12% more patients in the orlistat group achieved 10% weight loss or more. This translates into a number needed to treat (NNT) of eight, i.e. eight patients would need to be treated with orlistat plus lifestyle changes for 1 year instead of lifestyle changes alone, for one additional patient to lose at least 10% of their baseline body weight. Four of these RCTs looked at weight maintenance in the second year and found that the initial difference in weight loss between orlistat and placebo was maintained, although both groups regained the same amount of weight.

Regarding secondary endpoints, orlistat was associated with statistically significant reductions in total cholesterol, low-density lipoprotein cholesterol, blood pressure, fasting plasma glucose, HbA_{1C}, BMI and waist circumference, although concentrations of high-density lipoprotein cholesterol were slightly lowered.

Large placebo-controlled trials have demonstrated an average weight loss at 1 year of 10% with orlistat, compared with 6% in the placebo group, where both groups took a 500–800-kcal reduced diet.[8,9]

The Orlistat Swedish Type 2 diabetes Study Group[10] also compared orlistat with placebo, in combination with a weight management programme, on weight loss and metabolic control in obese type 2 diabetic patients. Orlistat induced significantly greater reductions in HbA_{1c} – 1.1% versus 0.2% – and fasting plasma glucose – 1.9 mmol/L versus 0.3 mmol/L.

A further study of 15 000 obese individuals demonstrated significant improvement in glycaemic control; 34% of diabetic patients were able to reduce or stop their diabetes treatment after taking orlistat with an average weight loss of 10.7%; 87% losing more than 5% of initial body weight and 51% lost over 10%.[11] Orlistat has also been shown to induce significant reductions in systolic (9.4 mmHg) and diastolic (7.7 mmHg) blood pressure compared with 4.6 mmHg and 5.6 mmHg on placebo.[14]

The XENDOS study[4] found that orlistat plus lifestyle changes produces a greater reduction in the incidence of type 2 diabetes than lifestyle modification alone. In this RCT, 3305 patients with a BMI of more than 30 kg/m^2, 79% with normal glucose tolerance and 21% with impaired glucose tolerance were randomised to lifestyle changes plus either orlistat or placebo for four years. At the end of the study period, the incidence of type 2 diabetes was 9.0% in the placebo group and 6.2% in the orlistat group and this equated to the number needed to treat (NNT) of 36. Yet it must be appreciated that these benefits only apply in patients with impaired glucose tolerance and that nearly half the patients in both groups failed to complete the study.

One message from the XENDOS study is that lifestyle changes are particularly effective in reducing the incidence of type 2 diabetes in overweight people with impaired glucose tolerance, and even more so in combination with the active agent. The NNT was 8, i.e. eight overweight people with impaired glucose tolerance (IGT) would need to undergo individualised lifestyle counselling for four years, to prevent one additional case of type 2 diabetes.

Individuals on orlistat can avail themselves of the MAP patient support programme, which provides advice and encouragement, and increases the likelihood of successful concordance and weight loss.

Side-effects

Adverse effects of orlistat are typically transient and usually affect the gastrointestinal tract. Unabsorbed fat is excreted in the faeces, leading to increased defecation, soft stools, oily discharge, flatulence and abdominal discomfort. The occurrence of side-effects is almost always the result of an inappropriately high dietary fat content, as with a low-to-moderate fat diet, effects are minimal. The existence of side-effects can be used to advantage, by demonstrating which foods have a high fat content, and should be avoided in the future.

Less than 1% of an oral dose of orlistat is absorbed. Orlistat does not alter the pharmacokinetics of digoxin, phenytoin, glibenclamide, alcohol, furosemide, captopril, nifedipine or atenolol but may interfere with absorption of ciclosporin. Absorption of fat-soluble vitamins (A, D, E and

K) may be decreased by orlistat and blood levels of these vitamins should be measured in patients taking the drug for more than 12 months.

Whereas concomitant use of orlistat does not affect the absorption of warfarin, there has been at least one case report in the US that noted clinically significant changes in INR associated use of orlistat. The only plausible explanation might be an effect on absorption of fat-soluble vitamin K, an essential component of blood clotting. Likewise there have been some concerns about the concomitant use of orlistat and the contraceptive pill. Again, if there is an effect it could be on absorption of the pill – there is no evidence for this – or on enterohepatic circulation.

Orlistat is known to affect the absorption of fat-soluble vitamins via inhibition of carboxylester pancreatic lipases. The effect of orlistat on vitamin and mineral absorption is of particular concern in the paediatric population, when growth and maturation are occurring. For this reason, many trials evaluating orlistat in adolescents monitored vitamin levels; some also evaluated mineral levels but none found a significant effect on the balance of key vitamins. This is possibly since the vitamins concerned are fat-soluble and obese individuals, including obese children, have ample stores of these vitamins in their livers. The use of orlistat in children should only be considered in specialist centres.

Contraindications

The drug is contraindicated in chronic malabsorption syndrome and cholestasis.

Sibutramine

Sibutramine (Reductil 10 mg and 15 mg capsules) inhibits noradrenaline and serotonin and, to a lesser degree, dopamine reuptake. It therefore has two simultaneous modes of action. Firstly, it acts centrally on hunger centres in the brain, leading to an early feeling of satiety and subsequent reduction in food intake. Effectively the 'start' signal to eat is unaffected, but the 'stop' signal is enhanced, usually allowing a person to be satisfied with two-thirds of their former customary intake. The enhanced satiety lasts long enough to discourage snacking or grazing. A degree of behavioural modification is crucial alongside drug treatment, as it is easy to override the lack of hunger, and rely on habit and other external cues to maintain calorific intake. The combination of sibutramine and behavioural therapy has been shown in trials to be more successful than either treatment modality alone.[13] Secondly, sympathetically mediated thermogenesis maintains basal metabolic rate (BMR) even when weight loss occurs. Normally, BMR will decrease as weight is lost, thus conserving energy and making it hard to lose more weight but this is theoretically avoided when using sibutramine.

The main evidence for the efficacy of sibutramine comes from the STORM study[7] which was designed to assess maintenance of weight loss in patients who initially respond to the drug. In the study, 605 individuals with a BMI of 30 kg/m^2 or more were given sibutramine 10 mg for 6 months, then those losing 5% or more of their body weight were randomised to either sibutramine or placebo. Lifestyle advice in both groups was based on 600 kcal fewer than requirements based on BMR and physical activity levels at baseline. Activity level, determined with the Baecke physical activity diary, and an extra 30 minutes walk per day was advised. The sibutramine group could increase to 15 mg or even 20 mg. A total of 467 patients achieved 5% weight loss in the initial 6 months and subsequently entered the randomised second phase. Of these, 43% of the sibutramine group maintained at least 80% of their weight reduction compared with only 16% of the placebo group. Weight loss in the sibutramine group was an average of 10.2 kg compared with 4.7 kg on placebo (although weight loss *per se* was not the point of the study). Furthermore, significant beneficial changes in cardiovascular risk factors occurred, including reduced triglycerides, markedly increased high-density lipoprotein cholesterol, reduced insulinaemia and C peptide levels, and decreased concentrations of uric acid. The study is a little difficult to interpret however, because the main effect of sibutramine is to restrict dietary intake by enhanced satiety, but this effect should theoretically be cancelled out by the closely defined lifestyle imposed upon both groups. STORM should therefore be underestimating the drug's efficacy.

A meta-analysis[7] assessed 10 RCTs (n = 2623) of sibutramine, two of which were in patients with controlled hypertension, and three of which were in patients with type 2 diabetes. Seven RCTs looked at the effects of sibutramine on weight loss at 1 year and found that patients lost 4.2 kg more than those taking placebo. Additionally 18–25% of patients achieved 10% weight loss or more at 1 year compared with placebo and the numbers needed to treat was six, i.e. for every six patients treated one achieved this level of weight loss.

Three RCTs assessed the effects of sibutramine in maintaining weight loss for up to 18 months and, in these three studies, between 10% and 30% more patients on sibutramine than placebo maintained at least 80% of their initial weight loss.[9]

NICE guidance

Use of sibutramine is endorsed by NICE and licensed for the management of obesity in adults between 18–65 years who have a BMI of 27 kg/m^2 or more, with one or more associated risk factors, or who have a BMI of

30 kg/m^2 or more. The starting dose is 10 mg daily with titration up to 15 mg after 4 weeks if no response is achieved. Therapy should be continued beyond 3 months only if the person has lost at least 5% of their initial body weight since starting treatment. Since the extent of initial weight loss in patients using sibutramine predicts the long-term response, it should be stopped if weight loss is less than 2 kg after 4 weeks on 15 mg. Treatment is not licensed beyond 12 months currently.

Side-effects

Common adverse effects of sibutramine include dry mouth, anorexia, insomnia, constipation and headache. Since sibutramine has been shown to increase blood pressure and pulse rate it is recommended that patients be monitored regularly throughout therapy. In clinical trials, systolic and diastolic blood pressure increased on average by 1–3 mmHg (including patients with hypertension controlled with a calcium-channel blocker with or without concomitant thiazide treatment) and pulse increased by approximately four or five beats per minute. However, results from the 6 week lead into the SCOUT (sibutramine cardiovascular outcomes) study suggest that patients who are normally contraindicated for treatment with the drug because of a history of cardiovascular disease showed falls in blood pressure and smaller increases in heart rate compared with the 'current labelled' population despite similar weight loss.[14]

Both blood pressure and pulse rate should be checked every 2 weeks for the first 3 months of treatment, every 4 weeks for the second 3 months, and then at least every 5 months after that. If an increase in heart rate of 10 beats per minute or a rise in blood pressure of at least 10 mmHg (systolic or diastolic) is found at two consecutive checks, therapy should be stopped.

Contraindications

Sibutramine is contraindicated in patients suffering from heart disease, congestive heart failure, cardiac arrhythmia or stroke. It should not be used in patients receiving monoamine oxidase inhibitors (MAOIs) or selective serotonin reuptake inhibitors (SSRIs) since the concomitant use of these drugs present the possibility of developing serotonin syndrome. This might be important when considering several over-the-counter OTC products that contain St John's wort. The drug is contraindicated in patients with major eating disorders or psychiatric illness.

Sibutramine is metabolised by the cytochrome P450 system and should be avoided in patients using erythromycin and ketoconazole since blood levels of these drugs will be altered.

Patients taking sibutramine can access the 'Change4Life' patient support programme.

Rimonabant

Rimonabant (Accomplia), a novel agent for obesity, works as a cannabinoid-receptor antagonist, blocking the CB_1 receptor. These receptors are located in the brain, gastrointestinal tract, adipose tissue, skeletal muscle, the liver and many other sites. The precise mechanism by which the CB_1 receptor is involved in energy balance is not known. Suggestions include reduction of appetite, diminished lipogenesis in adipose tissue and increased glucose uptake by muscle cells. Its ability to raise adiponectin levels, in particular, makes it a fascinating compound. Rimonabant is metabolised mainly in the liver, and excreted predominantly in faeces, with around 3% excreted in the urine.

It has been known for some time that recreational users of cannabis are commonly subjected to bouts of intense hunger and as a result they tend to overeat, a condition known as the 'munchies'. This side-effect of cannabis use alerted researchers to the possibility of blocking a common hunger mechanism by producing a drug that would act as a blocker on the CNS cannabinoid receptors. This proved to work and rimonabant was the first licensed agent from this area of research, yet that licence was suspended by the European Medicines Agency (EMEA) in November 2008 because of concerns about side-effects.

Rimonabant is effective in bringing about weight loss in obese individuals and a number of systematic reviews and meta-analysis support this. Rimonabant has additional benefits on lipid profile and glycaemia that are greater than would be expect by weight loss alone. In addition to reducing weight and waist circumference rimonabant also affects serum lipid levels in a positive way. In some studies mean weight loss after year 1 was 6.3 kg compared with 1.6 kg with placebo; 48% of patients on rimonabant lost at least 5% of body weight and 25.2% lost at least 10% of body weight. Comparable figures for placebo were 20% and 8% respectively. Using this data, the NNT works out at 5.[17] Continued use of rimonabant in the second year kept this weight loss while those randomised to placebo in the second year regained most of their lost weight. Using rimonabant, participants lost an average 6.1 cm of their waist circumference measurement compared with 2.5 cm with placebo. In addition, concentrations of high-density cholesterol rose by 12.6% in the rimonabant treated group, compared with 5.4% in the placebo group and triglycerides deceased by 5.3% compared with a 7.9% rise in the placebo group.[15]

Looking at secondary endpoint data, taking rimonabant is associated with statistically significant reductions in waist circumference, blood pressure and triglyceride concentrations, as well as increases in high-density lipoprotein cholesterol. High-density lipoprotein levels were unaffected, but a decrease in highly atherogenic, small, dense particles is demonstrated, in favour of particles with less dangerous characteristics. Statistically significant reductions in fasting blood glucose and HbA_{1c} concentrations were also seen in the RCT of patients with type 2 diabetes.[15] In drug-naive patients with diabetes, HbA_{1c} was reduced by up to 1.9%.[16]

There are currently no published studies of rimonabant looking at whether patients are likely to live longer or better with the drug, and the CRESCENDO study, which was looking at its effects on myocardial infarction, stroke and cardiovascular death over 5 years has been abandoned. Following suspension of the licence, Sanofi-Aventis, the drug's licence holder, announced that it was discontinuing the entire ongoing rimonabant clinical development programme.

Patients taking rimonabant certainly lost more weight over 12 months than those taking placebo by an average of 4.7 kg. Those receiving rimonabant were about five times as likely to achieve at least 10% weight loss than those taking placebo.[7]

Indication

Rimonabant, before the licence suspension, was indicated as an adjunct to diet and physical activity. It was licensed for managing obesity in adults who have a BMI of 27 kg/m² or more with one or more associated risk factors, or who have a BMI of 30 kg/m² or more. Dosage was 20 mg daily before breakfast and the drug was licensed to be used for more than 2 years as long as an individual decision was made with each patient at that time.

Side-effects

Patients with 'serious mental illness' were excluded from using the drug yet despite this, the drug has a relatively high incidence of psychiatric adverse effects. The 'depressive mood changes' the drug induced were primarily mild, including irritability and boredom, which were often deemed acceptable by patients. Rare severe side-effects had been minimised by the change in the SPC but included possible suicide ideation. A number of studies now support the concern that the frequency of psychiatric side-effects associated with use of this drug is greater that was initially thought. Data from 4105 participants in four trials comparing rimonabant 20 mg daily with placebo were examined.[17] Participants given rimonabant were 40% more likely to report adverse events, usually gastrointestinal disturbance or serious adverse events than patients given placebo.

This concern was always there. In July 2007 the Medicines and Healthcare Regulatory Products Agency in the UK issued a statement on the risk of psychiatric reactions in patients prescribed rimonabant. It noted that in clinical trials, depressive disorders or mood alterations with depressive symptoms have been reported in up to 10% of patients and suicide ideation in up to 1% of patients and that this risk may be increased in patients with a past history of psychiatric illness. Based in these findings, the SPC for the product was modified particularly to restrict its use in patients who have any form of depressive illness and to ensure improved monitoring by doctors for occurrence of depressive symptoms.

Then the European Licensing Agency (EMEA) suspended rimonabant's marketing authorisation at the end of October 2008 after a review concluded that the drug's benefits 'do not outweigh the risks of psychiatric reactions in clinical use'. Studies that had been completed since the product's initial approval show that there was approximately a doubling of the risk of psychiatric disorders in patients taking rimonabant compared with patients on placebo. New data from ongoing studies and from spontaneous reports of adverse effects from rimonabant suggested that serious psychiatric disorders, including depression, sleep disturbances, anxiety and aggression might be more common in clinical trials completed before licensing.

Contraindications

Rimonabant was contraindicated in patients with a history of mental health problems, including major depression, or those on antidepressant medication, and careful screening of patients, and a full explanation of potential side-effects was mandatory. However following changes in the SPC and in guidelines to tighten up prescribing safety, rimonabant was being used successfully in many patients in controlling their weight, helping reduce HbA_{1c} and avoiding insulin conversion. For many people rimonabant had been the only successful agent for weight loss. As NICE specified that rimonabant was to be used only after orlistat and sibutramine, there are no agents to replace it. Its withdrawal by the EMEA rather than limiting its use to specialist centres, or accredited prescribers in a similar way to Roaccutane (isotretinoin) represents a gross over-reaction, especially as it used mostly the same information that NICE had used in giving it a highly positive appraisal. It must be hoped that despite the current pessimistic situation that something will happen to allow its re-emergence in the future.

Rimonabant was not recommended in pregnancy and was contraindicated in breastfeeding. Caution was required in patients with moderate hepatic impairment and it was not recommended in patients with severe hepatic or severe renal impairment.

Combination drug therapy

According to NICE, combinations of anti-obesity drugs should not be used until efficacy and safety is established. Where mechanisms of action do not overlap, in theory combining drugs might result in additive weight loss. However, results from two clinical trials with orlistat and sibutramine suggest that this may not be the case.

Use in adolescents

Since children and young adults are also involved in the obesity epidemic there has been consideration on the use of pharmacological agents in the management of adolescent obesity. However, safety concerns and a lack of data restrict use in this patient group.

Orlistat is the only anti-obesity medicine approved for use in adolescents between the ages of 12 and 16 years. The most frequently reported adverse effects of orlistat in this patient group and in common with adults, were gastrointestinal; reduced concentrations of fat-soluble vitamins were also observed. Of the 6 clinical trials published, 5 have shown statistically significant reductions in body mass index (BMI) from baseline, ranging from 0.55 to 4.09 kg/m^2; one small trial failed to demonstrate significant weight reduction compared with placebo. Sibutramine has also been evaluated for use in overweight adolescents in six trials. Trials demonstrated a statistically significant reduction in BMI of up to 5.6 kg/m^2 (from baseline). Of concern is evidence indicating that sibutramine therapy may be associated with elevated blood pressure, increased pulse rate, depression, and suicidal ideations.[18]

Other pharmacological agents

With a potentially enormous market for therapeutic agents licensed for the management of obesity, many companies are seeking opportunities for their products. Many pharmaceutical agents such as zonisamide, bupropion or exenatide have been linked to or associated with weight loss and may be licensed for the management of obesity. A naltrexone-bupropion combination has been noted to reduce the prevalence of metabolic syndrome, improving cardiometabolic markers in high-risk subjects. Current research in diabetes has developed a number of pipeline products, which eliminate the weight gain caused by many hypoglycaemic agents especially insulin, sulphonylureas and thiazolidinediones.

The dipeptidyl peptidase-4 inhibitors sitagliptin and vildagliptin are weight neutral and the glucagon-like peptide mimetics, such as exenatide, induce very significant weight loss. Members of this class, in particular liraglutide, are likely to be licensed as obesity treatments. Pramlintide is a combination of amylin and leptin, and is injected alongside insulin to attenuate the associated weight gain. Sodium–glucose transporters (SGLT-2s) are under investigation as glycosuric agents in diabetes, and an obesity vaccine based on ghrelin antibodies is planned. However, other medicines show promise and the possibility that their use in obese patients, or in specific groups of obese patients such as those with type 2 diabetes, merit further consideration and investigation. These drugs include metformin, topiramate, tesofensine and lorcaserin.

Metformin

Metformin has been known to induce weight loss in obese patients for many years yet studies of long duration in obese patients are relatively scarce. The effect of metformin on body weight in RCTs in patients suboptimally controlled by diet was found to be variable.[19] About half of these studies demonstrate significant reductions in body weight with metformin relative to baseline or comparator agents. The longest treatment duration was the 10-year follow up of metformin-treated overweight patients in the UK Prospective Diabetes Study (UKPDS).[20] Patients receiving diet-based treatment gained about 2 kg over the course of the trial, with a slightly smaller weight gain of about 1.5 kg in the metformin group. The addition of metformin to sulphonylurea treatment in a subgroup of patients in this trial did not result in a significant weight change.

A number of studies have looked at the use of metformin in non-diabetic obese or abdominally obese subjects[20] and have shown a moderate effect in supporting weight reduction.

A randomised trial of 150 women with a BMI of more than 30 kg/m^2 (of whom 15 had type 2 diabetes) evaluated sibutramine, metformin or orlistat for 6 months.[21] Weight, waist and BMI were reduced in all groups (p < 0.0001) supporting the efficacy of metformin in the management of obesity.[22] A small, 7-month study in non-diabetic overweight patients (BMI >28 kg/m^2)[23] or morbidly obese subjects (mean BMI 43 kg/m^2)[24] demonstrated decreases in body weight with metformin, although only the latter study demonstrated a reduction in waist circumference.

An uncontrolled, retrospective analysis followed the progress of 26 women with hyperinsulinaemia and progressive weight gain refractory to diet and exercise who received a 1-year intervention of metformin together with a hypocaloric diet.[25] All but one of these patients lost 5% or more of initial body weight at 6 months, and 21 patients lost more than 10% of initial body weight at 12 months. Longer-term (2–4 years) follow up of 21 of these women demonstrated weight maintenance in 19 women with the final body weight correlating strongly with the initial weight loss during the original 1-year intervention.

Metformin may influence body fat distribution in patients with type 2 diabetes uncontrolled by diet. A post-hoc analysis from a randomised study of 26 weeks' duration showed that metformin significantly reduced visceral fat mass versus placebo whereas rosiglitazone did not.[26]

The effects of metformin on body weight are variable between patient populations. It is clear, however, that metformin does not increase body weight, in contrast to other oral hypoglycaemic agents, and may help to limit the weight gain associated with insulin- or sulphonylurea-based regimens. The improvements in glycaemia and clinical cardiovascular outcomes demonstrated for metformin are independent of changes in body weight or adiposity. This observation supports current recommendations relating to the suitability of metformin for initiation of oral anti-diabetic pharmaco-therapy in patients with type 2 diabetes, irrespective of body weight. There is no compelling evidence for the use of metformin to control body weight in non-diabetic populations.

Ren-Rong and his colleagues working in China[27] looked at the efficacy of lifestyle intervention and metformin alone and in combination, for anti-psychotic-induced weight gain and abnormalities in insulin sensitivity.

They designed a randomised, controlled trial involving 128 adult patients with schizophrenia in a mental health institute in China. Participants who gained more than 10% of their pre-drug weight were assigned to one of four treatment groups: 12 weeks of placebo, 750 mg per day of metformin alone, 750 mg per day of metformin and lifestyle intervention, or lifestyle interven-tion only.

Main outcomes measured in the study included: body mass index (BMI), waist circumference, insulin levels and insulin resistance index.

Where patients maintained relatively stable psychiatric improvement, the lifestyle-plus-metformin group had mean decreases in BMI of 1.8 kg/m². The metformin-alone group had mean decreases in BMI of 1.2. The lifestyle-plus-placebo group had mean decreases in BMI of 0.5 kg/m². The lifestyle-plus-metformin treatment was significantly superior to metformin alone and to lifestyle-plus-placebo for weight, BMI and waist circumference reduction.

Topiramate

In a multicentre, double-blind, placebo-controlled trial all subjects received a non-pharmacological programme of diet, physical activity and behavioural modification throughout the study; the assigned diet was 600 kcal per day less than the subject's individually calculated energy expenditure. After a 6-week single-blind placebo run-in, subjects were randomised to placebo, topiramate 96 mg per day or topiramate 192 mg per day. Following an 8-week titration period, subjects remained on their assigned dose for 52 weeks.[27]

Subjects in the placebo, topiramate 96 mg per day and topiramate 192 mg per day groups lost 1.7%, 4.5% and 6.5% respectively, of their baseline body weight and had absolute decreases in HbA_{1c} of 0.1%, 0.4% and 0.6% and the topiramate-treated subjects also experienced statistically significant decreases in systolic blood pressure. Most common adverse events were paraesthesia and events related to the central nervous system. Topiramate therefore appears to be effective for weight reduction and improvement in glycaemic control in obese subjects with type 2 diabetes treated with metformin monotherapy, and these results would suggest further investigation but it should be remembered that the drug is associated with negative effects on cognition and this would need to be taken into account.[28]

Qnexa is a pipeline product (a drug under investigation) containing low doses of phentermine and topiramate. In Phase II trials it achieved significantly greater weight loss than placebo and also each of the active single agents. The proportion of patients achieving over 10% body weight loss with Qnexa was greater than the sum of both active comparator agents.

Tesofensine

Tesofensine inhibits the presynaptic uptake of the neurotransmitters noradrenaline, dopamine and serotonin in the brain and was studied in patients with Parkinson's and Alzheimer's diseases, some of whom were obese and who recorded an unintended weight loss during treatment. The drug appears to work by suppressing hunger, leading to an energy deficiency that resulted in the burning off of excess body fat.[29]

In trials, tesofensine induced an average weight loss of 12.8 kg; 10.6% of body weight on 1 mg and 11.3 kg on 0.5 mg, equating to 9.2% of body weight. A 0.25 mg dose induced an average loss of 6.7 kg, 4.5% of body weight. The placebo group lost 2.2 kg, 2% of body weight.

The most common adverse events caused by tesofensine were dry mouth, nausea, constipation, hard stools, diarrhoea and insomnia. A key finding was that a dose of 0.25 mg daily and 0.5 mg daily showed no significant increases in systolic or diastolic blood pressure compared with placebo but heart rate was increased in the 0.5 mg daily group.[30]

Lorcaserin

Lorcaserin is selective in stimulating the 5-HT_{2C} serotonin receptor, located in the hypothalamus, which helps regulate satiety and influences metabolic rate. Results from a Phase II study demonstrate that treatment with lorcaserin produced highly statistically significant, progressive and dose-dependent weight loss over a 12-week period. In the study, which excluded diet and exercise, patients taking a daily 20 mg dose of lorcaserin recognised a mean weight loss of 3.0 kg, while patients on placebo lost less than 0.5 kg. Lorcaserin was generally well tolerated at all doses and had no apparent effects on heart valves or pulmonary artery vasculature.

The drug, in early 2009, was being assessed in a Phase III study, the BLOOM (Behavioral Modification and Lorcaserin for Overweight and Obesity Management) study. This double-blind, randomised, and placebo-controlled trial includes about 100 centres in the US, and is expected to enrol approximately 3000 overweight and obese patients. The proportion of patients with a 5% or greater weight reduction from baseline at week 52 is the primary endpoint.

References

1. Dixon J B. Weight loss medications – where do they fit in? *Aust Fam Phys* 2006; 35: 576–57.
2. National Institute of Health and Clinical Excellence. *Obesity Guidance on the Prevention, Identification, Assessment and Management of Overweight and Obesity in Adults and Children.* NICE Clinical Guidance CG43. London: NICE, 2006.
3. Van Gaal L F *et al.* for the RIO-Europe Study Group. Effects of the cannabinoid-1 receptor blocker rimonabant on weight reduction and cardiovascular risk factors in overweight patients: 1-year experience from the RIO-Europe study. *Lancet* 2005; 365: 1389–1397.
4. Gerstein H *et al.* Conference Report: International Diabetes Federation 19th World Diabetes Conference, Cape Town, 5 Dec 2006. Brussels: IDF, 2007.
5. Torgerson J S *et al.* Xenical in the prevention of diabetes in obese subjects (XENDOS) study: a randomised study of orlistat as an adjunct to lifestyle changes for the prevention of type 2 diabetes in obese patients. *Diab Care* 2004; 27: 155–161.
6. Christensen R *et al.* Efficacy and safety of the weight-loss drug rimonabant: a meta-analysis of randomised trials. *Lancet* 2007; 370: 1706–1713.
7. Rucker D *et al.* Long term pharmacotherapy for obesity and overweight; updated meta-analysis. *BMJ* 2007; 335: 1194–1199 and *BMJ* doi:10.1136/bmj.39385.413113.25 (online publication 15 Nov 2007).
8. James W *et al.* Efficacy of sibutramine on weight maintenence after weight loss: a randomised trial: The STORM Study Group. *Lancet* 2000; 356: 2119–2125.
9. Sjostrom L *et al.* Randomised placebo-controlled trial of orlistat for weight loss and prevention of weight regain in obese patients, European Multicentre Orlistat Study Group. *Lancet* 1998; 352: 167–172.
10. Davidson M H *et al.* Weight control and risk factor reduction in obese subjects treated for 2 years with orlistat – A randomized controlled trial. *JAMA* 1999; 281: 235–242.
11. Berne C. A randomized study of orlistat in combination with a weight management programme in obese patients with type 2 diabetes treated with metformin. *Diabetic Med* 2004; 22: 612–618.
12. Wirth A. Reduction of body weight and co-morbidities by orlistat: The XXL–Primary Health Care Trial. *Diabetes Obes Metab* 2005 Jan; 7: 21–27.
13. Bull E. Obesity: orlistat. *Drugs Context* 2004; 1: 193–232.
14. Wadden T, Stunkard A, eds. *Handbook of Obesity Treatment.* London: Guilford Press, 2002.
15. Pi Sunyer F *et al.* Effect of rimonabant, a cannabinoid-1 receptor blocker, on weight and cardiometric risk factors in overweight and obese patients; RIO- N America: A randomised controlled trial. *JAMA* 2006; 295: 761–775.

16. Maggioni A P *et al.* Tolerability of sibutramine during a 6-week treatment period in high-risk patients with cardiovascular disease and/or diabetes: a preliminary analysis of the Sibutramine Cardiovascular Outcomes (SCOUT) Trial. *J Cardiovasc Pharmacol* 2008; 52: 393–402.
17. Lawrence J. Warning over weight-loss drug. *The Independent*, 16 Nov 2007, 6.
18. Dunican K *et al.* Pharmacotherapeutic options for overweight adolescents. *Ann Pharmacother* 2007; 41: 1445–1455.
19. Golay A. Metformin and body weight. *Int J Obes* 2008; 32: 61–72.
20. UK Prospective Diabetes Study Group. Effect of intensive blood glucose control with metformin on complications in overweight patients with type 2 diabetes (UKPDS 34). *Lancet* 1998; 352: 854–865.
21. Gokcel A *et al.* Evaluation of the safety and efficacy of sibutramine, orlistat and metformin in the treatment of obesity. *Diabetes Obes Metab* 2002; 4: 49–55.
22. Pasquali R *et al.* Effect of long-term treatment with metformin added to hypocaloric diet on body composition, fat distribution, and androgen and insulin levels in abdominally obese women with and without the polycystic ovary syndrome. *J Clin Endocrinol Metab* 2000; 85: 2767–2774.
23. Mogul H R *et al.* Metformin and carbohydrate-modified diet: a novel obesity treatment protocol: preliminary findings from a case series of nondiabetic women with midlife weight gain and hyperinsulinemia. *Heart Dis* 2001; 3: 285–292.
24. Ramachandran A *et al.* The Indian Diabetes Prevention Programme shows that lifestyle modification and metformin prevent type 2 diabetes in Asian Indian subjects with impaired glucose tolerance (IDPP-1). *Diabetologia* 2006; 49: 289–297.
25. Wenying Y *et al.* The preventive effect of acarbose and metformin on the progression to diabetes mellitus in the IGT population: a 3-year multicentre prospective study. *Chin J Endocrinol Metab* 2001; 17: 131–135.
26. Ren-Rong *et al.* Lifestyle intervention and metformin for treatment of antipsychotic-induced weight gain. *JAMA* 2008; 299: 185–193.
27. Toplak H *et al.* Efficacy and safety of topiramate in combination with metformin in the treatment of obese subjects with type 2 diabetes: a randomized, double-blind, placebo-controlled study. *Int J Obes* 2005; 31: 138–146.
28. McElroy S *et al.* Topiramate in the treatment of BEDS associated with obesity. *Am J Psychiatr* 2003; 160: 255–261.
29. Astrup A *et al.* Weight loss produced by tesofensine in patients with Parkinson's or Alzheimer's Disesae. *Obesity* 2008; 16: 1363–1369.
30. Astrup A *et al.* Effect of tesofensine on bodyweight loss, body composition, and quality of life in obese patients: randomised, double-blind, placebo controlled trial. *Lancet* 2008; 372: 1906–1913.

12

Bariatric surgery

For some obese individuals, lifestyle advice and behavioural support with the addition of drug treatment will fail to achieve a reduction in BMI and as a result these individuals will remain at high risk of disease and early death as well as significant disability. For such individuals, neither lifestyle solutions nor pharmacotherapy will adequately address the problem and surgery to remove excess fat becomes an option. The term *bariatric surgery* collectively describes the surgical procedures intended to induce weight loss directly, and which are used in the management of obesity and its co-morbidities. Bariatric procedures can prove highly clinically effective, and also cost-effective, and may achieve long-term sustained weight loss and consequent improvement in health and global risk. The surgical management of obesity is a crucial, and increasingly prevalent facet of weight management, and in many people is the only effective method by which a sufficient quantity of weight can be shed. The latest advances in surgical techniques have produced safer, more effective and more cost-effective operations, so although the surgical option is still limited to a relatively modest number of extremely obese patients, for such people it is a vital method of improving health and quality of life.

Does surgery work and is it safe?

There now exists compelling evidence that surgery provides medically significant weight loss over time.[1] A group of nearly 8000 obese patients who had undergone gastric bypass surgery were compared with matched controls for age, gender and BMI. Follow up for an average of 7.1 years showed that those in the surgery group were 25% less likely to have died. A second study followed 14 000 patients after two bariatric surgical procedures and found that there was a mean loss of 53% of excess weight for vertical banded gastroplasty and a 72% mean loss for gastric bypass surgery.[2]

There will be a trade off between the risks of surgery and the consequences of lifelong obesity and associated complications. Yet the risks associated with bariatric surgery have decreased in recent years, especially with the advent of laparoscopic techniques that have reduced tissue injury and complications, particularly wound problems.[3] It is important to remember that following surgery – although diabetes is usually resolved, other risk factors are markedly reduced and premature death is significantly reduced compared with placebo – overall mortality risk, especially cardiovascular disease risk, is still greater than the background population. Individuals who have undergone bariatric surgery have a greater risk, at any given weight than their counterparts who have not undergone surgery, so they should be treated as high risk for cardiovascular disease for the rest of their lives, in terms of aspirin prescribing, blood pressure control, etc.

Who gets surgery?

Patients with morbid obesity were originally identified as being eligible for bariatric surgery using the criteria drawn up by the 1991 US National Institutes of Health (NIH) Consensus Conference Statement on Gastrointestinal Surgery for Severe Obesity.[4] This group of patients constituted those with a BMI of 40 kg/m^2 or more, or a BMI of 35 kg/m^2 or more in the presence of high-risk co-morbid conditions and these criteria are still widely recognised and accepted. Other authorities use a broader definition – a strictly weight-based definition is sometimes not appropriate, and a better definition of morbid obesity includes patients who have direct, weight-related serious morbidity, such as mechanical arthropathy, hypertension, type 2 diabetes, lipid-related cardiac disease and sleep apnoea.

The National Institutes of Health guidelines[4] for selecting patients for obesity surgery state that ideal candidates are people who:

- have failed attempts with non-surgical means of weight loss for at least 5 years and who are more than 100 pounds (45 kg) overweight or twice their ideal weight.
- fully understand the importance of the proposed surgical procedure, including all known and unknown risks.
- are willing to be observed for a prolonged period of time.
- have attempted weight reduction using conservative treatments without success. Documentation of such attempts will need to be provided at the time of consultation; if unavailable, a medically supervised weight reduction programme may be recommended before bariatric surgery is considered.

Contemporaneous data provided by the Scottish Obese Subjects Study[5] showed that surgery was superior to other approaches to obesity management, demonstrating better improvements in a range of indicators. On the social front there was an improvement in quality of life and this linked to the better chance of getting back into employment. Importantly, there was an overall reduction in the cost of healthcare in the surgery group. On the clinical side there were huge improvements: reductions in symptoms of type 2 diabetes, reduced blood pressure and fewer cases of hypertension, as well as other clinical parameters.

At that time, the Scottish Intercollegiate Guidelines (SIGN) suggested that surgery was the most effective treatment for selected patients with morbid obesity and recommended that surgery be carried out more frequently.[6]

Recently, in the UK however, the National Institute for Health and Clinical Excellence (NICE) has issued guidance that supersedes the NIH and SIGN guidelines.[7] NICE guidelines are summarised in box 12.1. It is estimated that in the fiscal year 2007–2008, the NHS funded around 3000 bariatric surgical operations. Prior to publication of the NICE guidelines, and for some time after publication, primary care trusts in England decided on an individual or group basis if they would or would not fund bariatric surgery and, if so, they decided on the criteria that would be used in selecting patients. For instance, the East of England Strategic Commissioning Group (ESCG) still insists on a BMI of 40 kg/m^2 or more, in addition to a confirmed diagnosis of type 2 diabetes or sleep apnoea treated with continuous positive airway pressure (CPAP). Northampton Primary Care Trust, however, follows NICE guidance to the letter. The benefit of such stringent criteria is to ensure that only the most needy patients, with co-morbidities such as diabetes or sleep apnoea, reap the benefits of scarce resources, and that everyone contemplating surgery has undergone first- and second-line therapies. Although this seems a sensible position to take, on the other hand, morbidly obese individuals with severe arthritis, non-alcoholic steatohepatitis and polycystic ovary syndrome, infertility or depression are wrongly denied surgery in direct, unethical and illegal contravention of NICE. Almost every area in the UK has unused capacity for bariatric surgery over and above the activity in which they are involved. For this reason access to surgery is poor, particularly on the NHS, and many patients resort to the private sector or head to Europe for surgery. However, when the NHS is allowed to undertake bariatric surgery on its patients, it provides a 'gold standard', state-of-the-art service, partly because of NICE's insistence on the provision of a multidisciplinary team approach, which weeds out inappropriate referrals, and because excellent preoperative and follow-up care is offered.

With publication of NICE guidance, primary care trusts are legally obliged to fund bariatric surgery for patients who meet the criteria (see box 12.1). Yet many trusts still agree funding on a case-by-case basis and the development across the NHS of specialist obesity services is proving to be a slow process.

Box 12.1 NICE guidelines for bariatric surgery under the National
Health Service

Bariatric surgery is recommended as a treatment option for adults
with obesity if all of the following criteria are fulfilled.

- The patient has a body mass index of 40 kg/m² or more, or
  between 35 kg/m² and 40 kg/m², and other significant disease
  (for example, type 2 diabetes or high blood pressure) that could
  be improved by weight loss.
- The patient has tried all appropriate non-surgical measures but
  has failed to achieve or maintain adequate, clinically beneficial
  weight loss for at least 6 months.
- The patient has been receiving or will receive intensive
  management in a specialist obesity service.
- The patient is generally fit for anaesthesia and surgery.
- The patient commits to the need for long-term follow up.

Bariatric surgery is also recommended as a first-line option (instead
of lifestyle interventions or drug treatment) for adults with a BMI of
more than 50 kg/m² in whom surgical intervention is considered
appropriate.

Health Trusts wishing to offer bariatric surgery have been required to
apply for 'preferred provider status'. In this application, evidence of a
multidisciplinary service, including physician, specialist nurse, dietician and
psychologist must be provided with evidence that preoperative assessment
will be undertaken. There must be evidence of the ability of the Trust to
provide the four main bariatric procedures and demonstrate how they will
support patients postoperatively.

Cost-effectiveness

Bariatric surgery is extremely successful in inducing long-term weight loss
because the intervention is considered to be (and almost always is) permanent, which dramatically reduces the risk of rebound weight gain. A successful procedure may induce a reduction of approximately 50–60% of excess
body weight, or a reduction in BMI of 10 kg/m² during the first 12–24
months postoperatively, therefore a person weighing 136 kg (300 pounds)
might realistically expect to achieve a weight loss of 45 kg (100 pounds).
The NHS Health Technology Assessment programme carried out an
economic evaluation of surgery for morbid obesity in 2002.[8] Surgery was
found to be more cost-effective compared with conventional treatment.

Despite the existence of formal guidelines that recommend bariatric surgery to be an appropriate procedure in cases of gross obesity (even in America, where surgery is relatively common compared with the rest of the world) in 2002, for example, only 0.6% of an estimated 11.5 million morbidly obese patients underwent the surgery. However, the numbers are increasing rapidly, demonstrated by a quadrupling of surgical procedures between 1998 and 2002 – from 13 386 to 71 733 – including a 900% rise in operations on patients between the ages of 55 and 64 years.[9]

The Swedish Obese Subjects (SOS) cohort study[10] is the best known study of bariatric surgery. It is a clinical intervention trial with long-term observation of patients undergoing weight loss by gastric banding, vertical banded gastroplasty or gastric bypass compared with those managed by conventional, non-surgical methods (figure 12.1). It began in 1987 and ultimately included over 4000 patients. The primary aim of the SOS study was to discover whether there is a reduction in total mortality with intentional weight loss; secondary aims were to examine the effects of weight loss on specific mortality and morbidity factors such as cardiovascular disease and diabetes, health-related quality of life and health economics.

Maximum weight reduction in all three of the surgical groups occurred after 1 year, which for the bypass group was approaching 40% of initial weight. Although some weight was regained by 10 years, the graphs for all surgical groups remain remarkably parallel to the control group. At 10 years, 74% of the patients in the gastric bypass group demonstrated a reduction of weight of greater than 20%. In contrast, a weight loss of less than 5% was shown in 73% of controls. The true benefits of the procedures are over and above weight loss however, and are evidenced by the corresponding

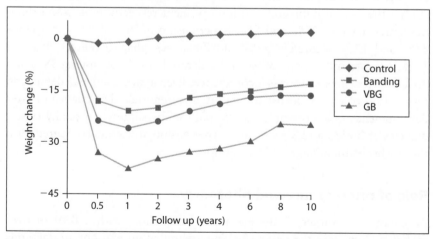

Figure 12.1 Swedish Obese Subjects cohort study. Ten-year follow-up of weight loss in controls on conventional obesity management and three different operative procedures. Reproduced from Ryden and Torgersen.[10]

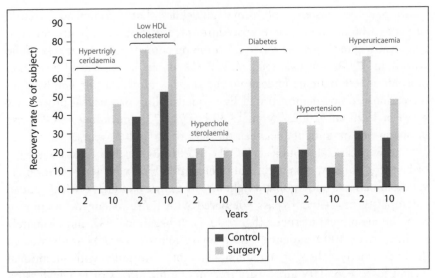

Figure 12.2 Swedish Obese Subjects cohort study. Likelihood of recovery from metabolic disturbances in the control group compared with the surgery group after 2 and 10 years. Reproduced from Ryden and Torgersen.[10]

cardiometabolic improvements. Figure 12.2 demonstrates the response of lipid profile, diabetes, blood pressure and gout to bariatric surgery.

Other trials have demonstrated more than 90% resolution rate of type 2 diabetes, two-thirds for hypertension, and improvements in high-density lipoprotein total cholesterol and triglycerides. Cardiovascular parameters including left ventricular wall thickness and left ventricular function improve as well as pulmonary function; sleep apnoea can disappear. In one study[11] the rate of remission and improvement respectively in co-morbidities were: diabetes 75% and 8%, hypertension 58% and 42%, dyspnoea 85% and 12%, arthralgia 52% and 24%, oesophageal reflux 79% and 11%, self-esteem 45% and 39%, and general physical functioning 58% and 33%. Improvements in stress incontinence, sleep apnoea, ankle oedema, and resumption of regular menstruation are also reported. The chance of later development of co-morbidities is also reduced by surgery; especially type 2 diabetes at both 2 and 8 years, and hypertension at 2 years compared with those who had non-surgical intervention.[7]

Role of primary care and pharmacy

Acceptance for surgery – the exception being those with a BMI of over 50 kg/m^2 – involves the patient having attempted all appropriate methods of weight loss, usually in the community setting, and then spending time under the auspices of a specialist obesity clinic. In the hands of such a clinic, they will expect to be assessed by a physician and seen by the multidisciplinary team of specialist nurse, psychologist and dietician, and may undergo a low-energy liquid diet in order to lose weight prior to surgery, and also to ensure that they can stick to the sort of liquid diet that is required 2 weeks before the operation, in order to shrink the liver, and in the immediate postoperative period.

Although many primary care professionals are aware of the use of bariatric surgery, others are not adequately informed about the referral criteria or preparation required and may know little about the latest techniques. So that although more referrals are now being made because of the greater interest in surgery, an increasing number are inappropriate. Because of the current increase in the prevalence of obesity, the burgeoning availability of surgery we are starting to witness, alongside the advent of quicker and cheaper laparoscopic techniques, coupled with the fact that surgical centres often have severely limited time for postoperative care, the role of primary care practitioners and pharmacy is assuming greater significance in providing preoperative, postoperative, medium- and long-term advice and support.

For some patients, albeit a small minority, bariatric surgery is the ultimate end point in the weight management process, which starts at the local slimming club, general practitioner or pharmacist. Anyone involved at any point along the weight-loss pathway must be aware of its existence, position and role, with special emphasis on the permanent nature of obesity surgery, and the complex nature of the aftercare, including the necessary vitamin supplementation, which includes vitamin B_{12} injections every 3 months. Each potential candidate for surgery will, by definition, be assessed, investigated and will undergo first-line management by diet, lifestyle changes, behavioural therapy and usually drug therapy before they are ready to discuss surgery. Primary care is ideally placed, having provided such initial treatment, to advise and to assist patients requiring referral onwards for consideration of surgery, by being aware which patients are suitable for surgery, and what the operative criteria are. They should have sufficient knowledge to be able to convey to a patient the realistic expectations of weight-loss surgery, and long-term postoperative care.

Cautions and contraindications

Although many patients fulfil the strict weight and co-morbidity criteria for bariatric surgery, there are patients who are unsuitable, and should be deselected before referral. These include patients with disordered eating, depression, low self-esteem and suicidal ideation, which must at least be diagnosed and treated before referral.

Binge eating is a relative contraindication to bariatric surgery, as is severe learning disability or cognitive impairment since such patients will be unable to eat and exercise postoperatively as required. For these reasons, severe mental illness is usually also considered to be a contraindication.

Women considering pregnancy are advised to delay surgery because of the rapid weight loss in the 12 months following surgery. Those who become pregnant will require close monitoring and vitamin supplementation, particularly supplementation of vitamins B_{12}, iron and folate. Studies have shown that babies born to mothers before bariatric surgery are more unhealthy and more prone to obesity than babies born to the same mother after surgery. Contraceptive advice is essential in women of child-bearing age, as fertility may be significantly increased immediately after surgery, because of rapid weight loss. Before surgery, an intensive assessment process must be adhered to, involving biochemical and endocrine screening, and psychological assessment. Schizophrenia, personality disorder and uncontrolled depression and other serious mental illnesses are absolute contraindications for surgery. Eating disorders such as binge-eating disorder and night eating syndrome should be managed prior to the consideration of surgery, and even so, may preclude surgery.

Preoperatively the risk–benefit ratio is carefully considered for every individual, and patients may be deemed unsuitable for surgery depending on their co-morbidities or anaesthetic risk. In major trials[7] the small number of deaths were due to surgical complications, and perioperative problems including subphrenic abscess (7%), pneumonia (4%), wound infection (4–6%), pulmonary complications (3–6%) and hepatic dysfunction (1.5%). In 2002, in-hospital death rates among patients undergoing weight-loss surgery were 0.32%, the death rate for men being three times higher than that for women.[7]

After surgery

The psychological implications of weight weight-loss surgery on an individual are immense, necessitating psychological assessment and counselling around their expectations of surgery, compared with the reality of what will actually occur, and whether they have the temperament and psychological stability to deal with the ramifications of surgery.

Some patients are so desperate to lose weight at any cost that they do not give much thought to 'life-after-surgery'. In the long term, after bariatric surgery the patient should be able to eat most foods without restriction. They will still enjoy the anticipation and preparation of food, and be hungry; they will enjoy eating, and feel full and satisfied afterwards. However, they will only be able to eat a few mouthfuls, before feeling satiated, while their companions continue eating. On a hot day, they will not be able to knock back a pint of water, but will have to drink it slowly. In a restaurant, they might only be able to eat a small proportion of an expensive meal, and then have to push the plate away. They will be able to eat more often, and will not be expected to go hungry, but their eating behaviour is changed forever.

For most people, these are the expected, and fiercely anticipated benefits of surgery, but for others, who have not adequately considered the ramifications of surgery, it can be a disaster. Different individuals have a different relationship with food, but a relatively high percentage of patients referred to specialist obesity clinics have an abnormal dependence on food. A person who reacts to stress, boredom, anger or depression by emptying the fridge, or demolishing a family-size bag of crisps, may be able to re-channel their emotions, but others may not be able to develop alternative coping strategies. To take away the ability to eat as a response to emotion can be disastrous in such people, who may either be unable to alleviate their underlying depression, or will develop dangerous alternative habits such as self-harm or addiction.

There are profound and permanent changes in store for anyone undergoing weight-loss surgery. It is the duty of both the primary and secondary care teams to anticipate these changes and prepare individuals as thoroughly as possible beforehand, and to provide care and support, both physically and psychologically after surgery. There may be problems for them in coming to terms with the loss of freedom to eat and drink anything that takes their fancy; to go out and enjoy a meal without restriction, and the possible unwanted side-effects of discomfort and vomiting. Most individuals will experience a change in body image, and often self-esteem, and the way they are viewed by their spouse, friends, relatives and the public. Some, especially women, may have gained weight as a way to avoid unwanted attention by the opposite sex, possibly due to some sort of abuse in the past: for them to lose weight and be the subject of compliments or wolf-whistles can be disturbing.

In pursuing the surgical option, an individual takes a major decision to surrender control of their weight to another person. While undergoing traditional treatment, a patient can still choose whether to turn up to Weight Watchers or not, whether to walk to work or take the car, whether or not to eat that last biscuit, or whether or not to take their weight-loss drug. Although they will still have to comply with healthy lifestyle advice after surgery, their last truly voluntary act of weight management is to sign the consent form for surgery and submit to the anaesthetic. Thereafter the surgeon assumes control, and a permanent change takes place; they will probably be physically unable to eat a meal above a certain size, or to eat certain foods without discomfort. For some patients, this handing over of responsibility amounts to an admission of failure, others view it as a great opportunity. Some individuals see it as a chance to deflect the blame onto someone else if they still do not lose sufficient weight.

Procedures

There are, historically, two categories of bariatric surgery procedures: restrictive and malabsorptive, used either alone or in combination. Malabsorptive procedures, or bypasses, were introduced in 1952 with the intestinal–jejunal bypass, whereas the restrictive gastroplasty techniques only began in 1971 with the horizontal gastroplasty. Malabsorptive surgery reduces the length of bowel through which the food passes, so that a smaller percentage of ingested food is absorbed from the gut. Postoperatively, patients may therefore eat what they please, but some nutrients will pass unabsorbed through the bowel. The most common example of malabsorptive surgery is the Roux-en-Y bypass.

Restrictive surgery works by reducing the size of the stomach to around the size of a golf ball so much smaller quantities of food can be ingested at any one time before a feeling of fullness and satiety is experienced. If excess food is eaten, discomfort, vomiting, regurgitation or bloatedness may develop. Examples of restrictive surgery include gastric stapling and laparoscopic gastric banding. Once food has passed through the restricted portion of the stomach it will pass normally through the rest of the bowel, so that nutrients consumed in the diet will become absorbed normally.

The jejuno-ileal bypass (figure 12.3) is now obsolete, and has not been performed since around 1980, however it is still just about possible that someone who had the operation in the 1970s or earlier may still present. In the operation, around 90% of the small bowel was bypassed by anastomosing the top of the jejunum to the end of the ileum, reducing the functional capacity of the bowel to only 45 cm, leading to rapid transit of food through the bowel, grossly inadequate digestion, malabsorption and steatorrhoea. The aim of allowing patients to eat and drink liberally without dietary

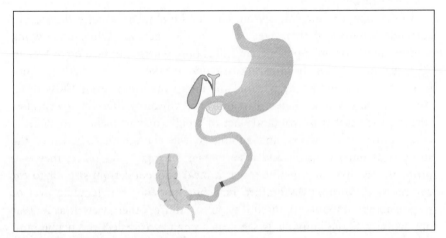

Figure 12.3 Jejuno-ileal bypass procedure.

restrictions, and still lose weight was successful, but at the expense of unacceptably severe, life-threatening complications and side-effects such as acute hepatic failure, cirrhosis, oxalate nephropathy and chronic renal failure, immune complex arthritis and malabsorption syndromes.

Gastric banding

Gastroplasty literally means 'changing the shape of the stomach' and has assumed a variety of incarnations. Initially it was performed by partitioning off a pouch of approximately 15–40 mL at the top of the stomach that filled rapidly with food, and emptied slowly through a narrow canal, like sand in an hour glass, into the body of the stomach. Thus the volume of food eaten was vastly reduced. Vertical banded gastroplasty is considered to be a forerunner to laparoscopic adjustable gastric banding (LAGB, figure 12.4), which involves an adjustable band being wrapped around the top of the stomach to reduce functional capacity.

The simplest and safest operation is laparoscopic placement of an inflatable band encircling the top 5% of the stomach to create a proximal 'pouch'. During follow up, saline is injected by a member of the surgical team, to inflate the band, which can later be adjusted by further injection or deflation to alter its tension restricting the passage of food, mainly solid food, to a greater or lesser extent. This is done through a permanent port, which is usually situated in the hypochondrium.

Side-effects

Surgical complications are seen in patients with LAGB. Discomfort or involuntary vomiting, or both, occur after poor chewing, rapid eating, exceeding pouch capacity or drinking shortly after eating. Interestingly, repeated

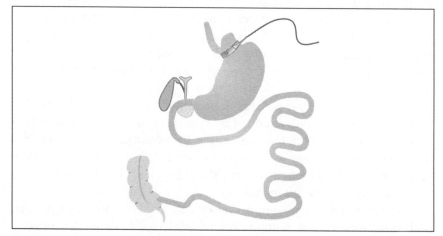

Figure 12.4   Laparoscopic adjustable gastric banding.

overeating or vomiting may cause the pouch to stretch, nullifying the initial restriction, allowing weight regain.

The subcutaneous port can occasionally cause prolonged discomfort and restrict movement. Band-related complications include band slippage or migration. This can be life threatening, requiring band replacement or removal. Nutritional deficiencies are rare but can occur if the band is too tight and the patient cannot eat properly. Death following surgery is rare and where it does occur, it is normally within 30 day of surgery; mortality risk is quoted at 0.1%. Overall 10–20% of patients do not achieve long-term weight loss with LAGB. Certainly motivation is required for successful weight loss with this technique.

Poorly motivated patients may encounter problems post-surgery. LAGB requires changing eating habits and appropriate adjustment of the band for optimal personalised restriction of food intake. Where the band is too loose, the patient may revert to his or her previous eating habits. If the band is too tight the patient may get around being able to tolerate solid foods by drinking high-energy fluids instead and thereby regain weight.

Patient motivation is essential for the success of LAGB. One study,[12] looking at which patients were more likely to benefit from this surgical intervention, found that those who were more likely to lose 50% of their weight:

- were aged 15–39 years
- had a BMI of 35–39 kg/m²
- were motivated to maintain an exercise regimen
- changed their eating habits.

Efficacy

People using gastric banding have been shown to lose a lot of weight, in one study on average 28.6 kg.[3] A further study showed that LAGB insertion of a gastric band resulted in patients losing 30–35 kg of their excess weight and maintaining that for at least 6 years.[13] One study has found that the cost of each kilogram of weight lost was less for surgical treatment than medical treatment, when examined over a 5-year period.[14]

This is impressive but perhaps more importantly, this weight loss has been associated with a resolution of existing type 2 diabetes in around 48% of patients. There was an improvement in hyperlipidaemia in around 59% of patients; hypertension was resolved in over 70% of patients and sleep apnoea was resolved or improved in 68% of patients. This surgery is clearly associated with significant improvement in clinical outcomes.

Compared with non-surgical interventions (very-low-energy diet, education, professional support, behavioural modification plus orlistat) patients with moderate obesity (BMI 30–35 kg/m²) who had a gastric band inserted lost on average 21% of their initial weight at 2 years compared with non-intervention subjects who lost 5.5% of initial weight.[3] LAGB can, however, be disappointing in those patients with very high BMIs.

Gastric bypass surgery

The Roux-en-Y gastric bypass divides the stomach to create a 20–30 mL gastric pouch, which is then stapled closed (figure 12.5). The remaining portion of the stomach, as well as approximately 90 cm of small bowel is bypassed. A Y-shaped portion of the small intestine is then attached to the pouch of the stomach and the obsolete section of stomach and bowel is re-anastomosed lower down the duodenum, to allow intrinsic factor and other proteins to re-enter the gut. This procedure is now routinely performed laparoscopically.

Efficacy

The procedure is effective, with a review of the current studies, involving over 7000 patients, reporting a mean weight loss of approximately 43.5 kg.[3] In addition this weight loss was associated with positive clinical outcomes; diabetes was resolved in 84% of patients, hyperlipidaemia was resolved in approximately 97% of patients, hypertension was resolved or improved in 87% of patients and sleep apnoea resolves or improved in approximately 95% of patients.

Side-effects

As with LAGB, surgical complications occur in around one-fifth of patients. There are slightly fewer reports of electrolyte balance and gastrointestinal

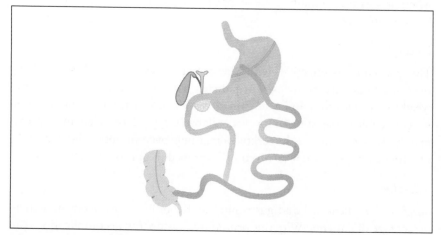

Figure 12.5 Gastric bypass surgery.

problems. The more common early complications include deep vein thrombosis, pulmonary embolism, leaks from anastomoses and staple lines, and later, inadequate weight loss and nutritional deficiency. Perioperative mortality is quoted as between 0.5 and 1%. Dumping syndrome (see below) occurs at one time or another in the majority of patients, caused by sugar entering the small bowel earlier, and becoming rapidly absorbed into the blood stream, accompanied by an insulin surge.

Indeed, late complications of the procedure include malabsorption problems such as anaemia and vitamin B_{12} and calcium deficiencies, although these are minimised by diligent vitamin and mineral supplementation, including lifelong B_{12} injections. Other potential complications include stoma stenosis, gastrointestinal haemorrhage and dumping syndrome, which is the rapid emptying of the stomach, leading to nausea, vomiting and bloating, cramping and diarrhoea as well as dizziness and fatigue.

Biliopancreatic diversion

More drastic forms of surgery exist for so-called 'superobese' individuals who have a BMI of over 50 kg/m², are 225% overweight or weigh more than 180 kg (400 pounds) with life-threatening obesity-related morbidity. These procedures involve resection of the distal 80% of the stomach, with gastro-ileostomy and diversion of biliary and pancreatic secretions to the distal ileum. Biliopancreatic diversion and long-limb gastric bypass leave less absorptive small bowel and in this way reduce obesity. Standard biliopancreatic diversion involves removing the lower third of the stomach and anastomosing the remaining stomach pouch to a portion of the small intestine to where the stomach was originally attached. A number of variations of this procedure exist. The procedure is technically difficult to perform and where it was traditionally done as open surgery, it is now often performed laparoscopically.

Efficacy

This procedure is effective, with a systematic review of studies, involving over 4000 patients, showing that patients with this procedure had a mean weight loss of around 46 kg.[3] Again, as with other procedures that reduced weight, clinical measures improved: diabetes type 2 resolved in approximately 99% of patients, hyperlipidaemia improved in approximately 99% of patients, hypertension resolved or improved in approximately 75%.

Side-effects

Surgical complications and gastrointestinal complications occur in a small percentage of patients. With this procedure, postoperative complications can be more severe. Malabsorption complications include fat being poorly absorbed resulting in steatorrhoea; flatus, foul-smelling stools, protein malnutrition, hypoalbuminaemia, anaemia, oedema, and alopecia. Patients will therefore require lifelong close monitoring of nutritional status and supplementation with calcium and vitamins.

Sleeve gastrectomy

Sleeve gastrectomy can be used as a first-stage procedure for patients who have a BMI of more than 50 kg/m² in order to induce weight loss before a second-stage gastric bypass procedure is considered, yet since it is often successful in its own right, it can be the sole procedure in a given patient.

Sleeve gastrectomy involves removing all but a narrow sleeve of the stomach, so that effectively the cylinder of the oesophagus joins a cylindrical stomach, with the greater curvature resected, which then joins the small bowel. It is therefore purely a restrictive procedure, and is often useful for individuals with excess weight, but who are otherwise healthy. It is a relatively simply and rapid procedure and can be achieved laparoscopically.

Miscellaneous surgical procedures

Following surgery, some patients are left with substantial folds of excess skin, which they may consider to be ugly. Apronectomy is a procedure used after dramatic weight loss to remove these overhanging folds of excess skin. It is not restricted to the abdomen – skin contouring operations include brachioplasty, and the inner and outer aspects of the thighs, and men may undergo pseudogynaecomastia correction. Unfortunately these procedures are rarely funded as part of the bariatric surgery programme, so can involve private treatment and cost.

Other surgical procedures have a limited or peripheral value in weight management. An artificial bezoar is a balloon which is inflated in the stomach, restricting its functional volume, and limiting food intake. It is sometimes used when immediate weight loss is urgent and critical, or to help patients reach a safe weight for more definitive bariatric – or indeed any – later surgery. It has no use in long-term programmes. Gastric pacing devices are being studied for their effects on weight loss; a laparoscopically implanted device is inserted into the stomach wall, in order to stimulate the nerves therein, to induce satiety in a patient.

Liposuction is a successful, purely cosmetic procedure, as it has no impact on cardiometabolic risk conferred by visceral fat. It involves suction of subcutaneous fat by way of a trochar resulting in the removal of up to 12 litres of fat in extreme cases.

Jaw wiring is an obsolete procedure, which even in its heyday caused only temporary weight loss.

Conclusion

Bariatric surgery offers the opportunity for considerable and permanent weight loss in individuals where other weight-loss strategies are found to be ineffective in reducing disease risk. The commonly used surgical procedures are relatively safe and cost-effective but is often seen as a last resort, with many local health authorities failing to comply with NICE guidelines in setting up multidisciplinary teams to support these surgical services or failing to provide sufficient funding. Patients who do submit for surgery need to be properly screened and supported, not only before and during the procedure but also postoperatively. Surgery will impose lifestyle changes to which some patients will find difficulty adapting, and therefore counselling services are required. Primary healthcare professionals, pharmacists and general practitioners need to appreciate the needs of patients considering surgery, so that appropriate advice and support can be given and ongoing monitoring assured.

References

1. O'Brien P *et al*. Treatment of mild to moderate obesity with laparoscopic adjustable gastric banding or an intense medical programme: a randomised trial. *Ann Intern Med* 2006; 144: 625–633.
2. Chapman A *et al*. Laparoscopic adjustable gastric banding in the treatment of obesity: A systematic literature review. *Surgery* 2004; 135: 326–351.
3. Anon. Surgery for obesity in adults. *Drug Ther Bull* 2008 Jun; 46: 41–45.
4. Maggard M A *et al*. Meta-analysis: surgical treatment of obesity. *Ann Intern Med* 2005; 142: 547–559.
5. Naslund L. Lessons from the Swedish obese subjects study: the effects of surgically induced weight loss on obesity co-morbidity. *Surg Obes Relat Dis* 2005; 1: 140–144.
6. Scottish Intercollegiate Guidelines Network. *Obesity in Scotland: integrating prevention with weight management*. Edinburgh: SIGN, 1996.
7. National Institute of Health and Clinical Excellence. *Obesity Guidance on the Prevention, Identification, Assessment and Management of Overweight and Obesity in Adults and Children*. NICE Clinical Guidance CG43. London: NICE, 2006.
8. National Institute for Health and Clinical Excellence. *Guidance on the Use of Surgery to Aid Weight Reduction for People With Morbid Obesity*. NICE Technology Appraisal Guidance. London: NICE, 2002.
9. Agency for Healthcare Research and Quality. *AHRQ Study Finds Weight-loss Surgeries Quadrupled in Five Years*. Press Release, July 12, 2005. Rockville, MD: Agency for Healthcare Research and Quality. http://www.ahrq.gov/news/press/pr2005/wtlosspr.htm (accessed 27 October 2009).
10. Ryden K, Torgersen A. In: *Surgery for Obesity and Related Diseases*. Vol 2, 2006: 549–556.
11. Avenell A *et al*. Systematic review of long-term effects and economic consequences for treatments for obesity and implications for health improvement. *Health Technol Assess* 2004; 8: 1–182.
12. Cotttam D *et al*. The impact of laparoscopy on bariatric surgery. *Surg Endosc* 2005; 19: 621–627.
13. Buchwald H *et al*. Bariatric surgery: a systematic review and meta-analysis. *JAMA* 2004; 292: 1724–1737.
14. Puzziferri N *et al*. Three year follow up of a prospective randomised trial comparing laparoscopic versus open gastric bypass. *Ann Surg* 2006; 243: 181–188.

13

Fad diets

The search for the dietary equivalent of the Holy Grail – a diet that allows rapid weight loss without effort or deprivation – has been largely fruitless and, taking into account human metabolism, seems likely to remain so. Yet, as a society, we are passionate in this quest and every year a new dieting sensation is unveiled to an increasingly gullible public. The search for a means of losing weight or preventing weight gain is big business. Entering obesity into a major search engine results in more than 35 million 'hits'; there are few health topics where there is greater media interest, conflicting advice, self-help manuals, popular myths, misinformation and unsubstantiated celebrity endorsements. Unlike medicines, the diet industry has little if any regulation and annually Americans spend a massive $33 billion on 'slimming' and in the UK the slimming industry was estimated in 2007 to be worth £11.2 billion.

Most adults in the United States adopt an energy-restricted diet at some time in their lives and the trend in the UK is similar. However, long-term success rates from individuals attempting to reduce body weight tend to be poor, with 50% of weight loss regained within 1 year. Losing weight is difficult and many are unsure or confused as to how to go about it effectively. It is therefore common for commercial interests, in response, to tout interventions that imply that weight loss can be obtained with minimal effort.

Wherever weight loss is offered to the public, the public respond in droves. Weight Watchers , the market leader in the UK, claims to have one million members. Self-help books that provide weight-loss strategies are often best sellers – *Dr Atkins' New Diet Revolution* has sold more than 10 million copies – and in recent years the internet has become an increasingly important conduit for weight-loss programmes.

Although commercial diets provide consumers with a plethora of choice, data on their comparative efficacy are limited. With little, if any, regulation in this market, it is confusing for the public, and in some cases healthcare professionals, to appreciate the relative merits, safety and efficacy of any specific programme.

Box 13.1 *Banting: the Atkins forerunner*

In 1862 William Banting, a London undertaker, consulted an ear, nose and throat specialist, Dr William Harvey, about his worsening hearing, which Harvey attributed to the bulk of fat compressing his airways, in other words, his obesity.

Harvey had recently returned from Paris where he had heard Dr Claude Bernard discuss a new theory of the role of the liver in diabetes. Bernard theorised that the liver, as well as secreting bile, also secreted a 'sugar-like substance' that it produced using elements of the blood passing through it.

Harvey considered the role of various foods as a cause of diabetes and began researching the physiology of fats, sugars and starches. A diet they came up with proved effective for Banting and in May 1863, at his own expense, he published the first edition of his pamphlet 'Letter on Corpulence'.

After 38 weeks, 66-year-old Banting had lost 46 pounds (21 kg) in weight and 12 inches (30 cm) off his waist. He lost nearly 1 pound (0.45 kg) per week from August 1862 to August 1863.

Banting claimed to never be hungry and apparently suffered no side-effects from the new diet.

He wrote: 'I can confidently state that quantity of diet may safely be left to the natural appetite; and that it is quality only which is essential to abate and cure corpulence.'

Historical background

'Diet' derives from the Greek word *diaita*, meaning 'way of life' and the science of dietetics has existed since the time of Hippocrates (c. 460–377 BC). Originally diet was merely that food which a person ate to stay alive – whatever was available. Later (many people say because of the teachings of Moses) diet became more complex, and was perceived to be the way to maintain health – some foods were considered good, and others bad. Only as the seeds of the current obesity epidemic were sown in the 19th century was it that 'diet' became synonymous with a means of losing weight and regaining health.

Special commercial diets for weight loss have been around for many years, perhaps as far back as the 1860s, when William Banting published a pamphlet as a response to his own dramatic weight loss (box 13.1). Banting's diet is held up as the forerunner to the Atkins diet, being low in 'farinaceous' food, or carbohydrate. There were important differences, however, such as Banting recommending 7 units of alcohol per day.

In 1909 Horace Fletcher gave his name to Fletcherism – a hugely popular weight loss method involving prolonged mastication of food, and spitting out the residue. At the same time, at the Battle Creek Sanatorium in the US, John Harvey Kellogg was becoming obsessed with bowels and predigested food both for weight loss and the maintenance of health, and in the process invented the cornflake.

The modern commercial application of dieting perhaps goes back to the Hays system in the early 1900s and later to *This Slimming Business* by John Yudkin and first published in 1958 (latest edition Penguin Books, 1970, op). Yudkin, a medical practitioner, qualified and applied a simple cause and effect – calories in/calories out – approach to weight loss, first recognised by Hippocrates. His approach was essentially a low-carbohydrate diet cutting down or cutting out bread, pasta, cereals, confectionary, cakes, biscuits, potatoes and alcohol and was based on the emerging work of Ansel Keyes, of the role of diet in heart disease. For many people it worked but for most, success was unsustainable.

Why fad diets can fail

Commercial diets are aggressively marketed, and claims made about their efficacy in inducing weight loss are not scientifically substantiated. Individuals who adopt these diets may lose weight, sometimes in large amounts, but this is normally regained within 12 months.

Overweight and obesity increase the risk of disease, therefore losing weight is encouraged by healthcare professionals as weight loss reduces this risk. Often the motivation for the individual is not health related but rather cosmetic, a wish to improve appearance. Ideally a weight-reduction programme will deliver both.

For most overweight and obese people, weight reduction can potentially be induced by a combination of an energy-deficient diet and increased exercise. Diets should always be balanced, containing the appropriate proportions of fat, carbohydrate, protein and minerals and vitamins. There has always been concern that 'fad' diets, even when they bring about weight loss, may not reduce health risk and may be associated with their own complications. Strict dieting involving the consumption of very few calories can be dangerous in the young, particularly teenage girls. One per cent of females aged 15–25 years have anorexia and bulimia that might have lifelong effects and in rare cases lead to death. Extreme dieting deprives the body of essential nutrients and can lead to excessive consumption of certain foods in unhealthy amounts. However, applying appropriate diet, activity and lifestyle measures early in life protects against both anorexia and obesity, eating disorders and disordered eating.

'Yo-yo' dieting, that is losing large amounts of weight over a short period of time but then regaining it again quickly, is damaging to health. As weight gain is an independent risk factor separate from excess weight, so the more pounds a person gains following repeated dieting is additive in terms of cardiometabolic risk. The weight loss/gain cycle may increase the risk of heart disease, myocardial infarction and premature death. Certainly if the weight is regained then any health benefit has been nullified and, worse still, it might be that the method of dieting employed might in itself be detrimental.

Buying diet aids (Chapter 14) or joining 'fad' diet groups can become a substitute for willpower and lifestyle change, especially if a normal, healthy weight is to be achieved and sustained. Some of the programmes can be spartan, subjecting the individual to constant hunger. Such hardship is only sustainable in the short term; when weight is lost, the fad diet is abandoned and the individual will regain the lost weight. When they fail they feel guilt and self-hatred.

Geoffry Cannon and Hetty Einzig[1] forcefully made these points in their book *Dieting Makes You Fat* (re-issued in 2008). This book, considered by some to be seminal, dissected the facts behind the failure of many commercial diets to support sustainable weight loss. It attempted to unmask the deficiencies in most weight-loss programmes using basic human metabolism as evidence for the prosecution, propounding a simple model that strongly supports the avoidance of processed foods and increasing physical activity.

All diets are designed to make users eat less and/or expend more energy. Some claim additionally to alter metabolism, to burn off calories faster or absorb them more slowly. But if there is any effect on metabolism, which is hotly disputed, then the effect is minimal.

The 10-potato diet

The unacknowledged principle behind many commercial or 'fad' diets is to make eating more difficult. Some require elaborate preparation or are unappetising or are bound by rigid rules. Cannon and Einzig[1] describe a diet created by Dr Denis Burkitt, Galway University, Republic of Ireland, who got volunteers to eat 10 large, baked potatoes in their skins every day for 3 months. Most lost weight as the 10-potatoes diet only created 1200 kcal, less than the daily energy requirement for males. Yet Burkitt allowed his volunteers to eat anything else they wished during the trial, so long as they ate the 10 potatoes. It seems the volunteers' lack of appetite caused by their consumption of potatoes supported their weight loss, rather than some metabolic stimulant present in the humble Irish potato. Cannon and Einzig cynically suggest that no one has yet become rich and famous on this 'Irish Diet'!

The ideal diet

The weight-reducing diet considered by many physicians and researchers as 'gold standard', is to eat 600 kcal less than a person's nutritional requirement – rather than their actual consumption – each day. This is equivalent to cutting out a Mars bar and a Danish pastry a day, and engaging in more activity than normal. This will result in sustained weight loss, and is healthy and manageable, if not very exciting.

The National Institute of Health and Clinical Excellence (NICE) has published recommendations for weight reduction and weight-loss programmes. NICE states that weight-loss programmes should only be recommended by healthcare professionals and funded within the NHS where they are based on a balanced healthy diet, encourage regular activity and aim to reduce weight by no more than 1 kg per week (ideally 0.5–1.0 kg).

The Office of Fair Trading (OFT) launched a campaign in November 2007 to persuade consumers not to buy 'miracle' diets. It suggested that 200 000 people in the UK each year spend a total of £20 million on diets that do not work. Women are the most frequently targeted. OFT advice to consumers is that they should disbelieve:

- claims that products offered by mail order or email contain 'special formulae'
- claims that scientific medicine has overlooked, or hidden scientific 'breakthroughs'
- testimonials from so-called satisfied customers.

OFT warns that 'scammers exploit people's desperation for a miracle cure. These diets are untested and may contain dangerous ingredients.' Fad diets, it seems, promise quick results with little effort, a promise that is hard to keep.

Popular slimming diets fall into a number of categories:

- high-fat, low-carbohydrate diets, e.g. the Atkins Diet, Lipotrim
- very-low-fat diets, e.g. the Ornish diet
- glycaemic index/load diets, e.g. the Glucose Revolution
- food-combining diets, e.g. the Hay System
- meal replacements, e.g. Slim-Fast
- miscellaneous, e.g. the Blood Type Diet, the Cabbage Soup Diet, the Beverly Hills Diet and the No-Diet Diet.

Although some of these programmes have evidence of long-term efficacy, and are scientifically validated, others are non-compliant with healthy eating principles. These may lead to weight loss in the short term, but they do not encourage the change in eating behaviour necessary for maintaining a lower weight.

Diet books and programmes

A bewildering plethora of commercial diets books and weight-loss programmes are aggressively promoted to the general public, who often find the concepts and claims behind the techniques tempting, although difficult to understand. An assessment of the more popular of these books and programmes follows. The term 'fad' diet might be regarded as a pejorative term and will be unacceptable to those who promote and support these diets. It is not intended to discredit any specific weight-loss programme and it is accepted that some individuals have successfully used specific weight-loss programmes and have succeeded in losing considerable amounts of body weight, which they have managed to keep off over time. However, it is important that all diets are viewed against current NICE guidance and are scientifically validated. Furthermore, the evidence base, where it exists, will be used to substantiate or otherwise the claims being made. Sadly this evidence base is often lacking.

Low-carbohydrate diets

Atkins Diet

Perhaps the most successful and most popular low-carbohydrate weight-loss diet is the *Dr Atkins New Diet Revolution*.[2] Dr Robert C Atkins published a number of books based on the same basic principle of a high-fat and low-carbohydrate diet. This weight-loss programme has the power to effect considerable weight loss in a short time.

Atkins works by restricting carbohydrate to less than 10% of energy consumed, so insulin secretion is suppressed. Without sufficient insulin, the body cannot metabolise glucose as a primary source of energy and in this circumstance two things happen. In the absence of insulin, glucagon, a hormone, is released and stimulates gluconeogenesis in the liver. In this way, over a week or two, the liver is depleted of its stores of glycogen and associated water molecules. Owing to such marked fluid loss, and associated diuresis, the resultant weight loss over the first week or two can be significant. This is the reason for the initial rapid loss of weight experience by those using the diet.

Additionally, subsequent to loss of its glycogen stores, the body metabolises fat, the end result of which is ketones – as it is in uncontrolled diabetes. The state of ketosis not only induces the trademark 'pear drop' smell on the breath, but also is an appetite suppressant. Data show that individuals following Atkin's method tend to benefit from greater weight loss at 6 months compared with those following different regimes, but after a year the extra benefit is lost, although the method has proven at least as good as its rivals.[3] However, it is an expensive diet, based as it is on meat, fish, eggs and cheese, and it lacks some essential dietary standards such as whole-grains, fruit and vegetables, erroneously promoting an increase in saturated fat. Furthermore, a protein-based diet can soon become unpalatable because of the lack of bread, pasta and other staple carbohydrates.

Research shows that people who stuck with the Atkins Diet for more than a year tended to have headaches, muscle cramps and diarrhoea caused by carbohydrate deficiency.[3] The minimum daily requirement of carbo-hydrate in adults is 150 g daily; Atkins restricts carbohydrates to 30 g daily.

Lipotrim

The Lipotrim programme is a popular weight-loss programme sold through pharmacies and other health food outlets. It is essentially a high-fat, low-carbohydrate diet. In the programme, the dieter is supplied with a range of prepared foods and vitamins that control the diet and ensure compliance to the high-fat, low-carbohydrate Atkins-type diet.

The South Beach Diet

Developed by Dr Arthur Agatston, an American cardiologist, and first published in 2003, *The South Beach Diet*[4] is very definite in its claim that it is 'not low carb'. But then 'it is not low fat either'. In reality it is a modi-fication of the Atkins diet, focusing on a staged approach to weight loss. In stage 1, the first 2 weeks, it is an Atkins-type diet focusing on high fat and strict exclusion of starches and sugars. There is a strong emphasis on the difference between 'good carbohydrates' (fibre and complex starches) and 'bad carbohydrates' (simple sugars and refined starches) and 'good fat' (essential fatty acids, polyunsaturated and monounsaturated fats) and 'bad fats' (saturated fats and trans fats). Dr Agatston uses his medical back-ground and credentials to persuade readers that consumption of only the 'good fat' and 'good carbs' is the way to lose weight and sustain a lower BMI. From a healthy-eating perspective, and once the initial weight-loss period is over, this could be considered to be an effective method of main-taining a nutritious diet. There is, however, no strong support for exercise in this diet. There is also to some degree a sense that the 'good' fats and carbs are likely to be linked directly to 'good' and 'bad' cholesterol, and this can be slightly misleading for those readers who do not appreciate the complex biochemistry and metabolism of fats.

The New High Protein Diet

First published in 2004 by Dr Charles Clarke, *The New High Protein Diet*[5] promises to allow readers to 'lose weight quickly, easily and painlessly'. It might be of some concern to public health specialists that it endorses the view that obesity 'is a medical problem and not just a problem of overeating'. In fact the author goes on to state that the overeating explanation for obesity 'is completely incorrect'. Despite the evidence to the contrary, he propounds a simple alternative explanation for the obesity epidemic: 'an imbalance of hormones'.

The programme promotes consumption of certain combinations of foods while avoiding others. In common with Atkins, the aim of this diet is to avoid stimulating insulin; everything containing refined carbohydrates is excluded. The diet is similar to Atkins in that access to a high-protein diet can only be gained through a high-fat diet, as the foods recommended include meat, poultry, fish, shellfish, cheese and eggs. Complex carbohydrates, such as those contained in vegetables, are allowed. In essence it is Atkins with complex carbohydrate flexibility. Like the South Beach Diet, there are stages to the New High Protein Diet. Stage 1 induces weight loss while carbohydrate intake is restricted to about 50 g per day, and fruit is totally restricted. In this stage, weight is lost quickly as in Atkins. Once target weight is reached, or when weight loss stops, the dieter moves to stage 2, where carbohydrates are reintroduced to a limited degree, mainly in the form of complex carbohydrates.

Low-carbohydrate and other ketotic diets can induce significant weight loss, and are an ideal solution for improving health for certain individuals. Evidence also demonstrates an improvement in cardiometabolic risk markers such as cholesterol, despite the nutritional changes. However, Atkins and other programmes are flawed because of the insistence on extra saturated fat within the regimen, alongside insufficient beneficial fruit and vegetables.

Various academic and clinical centres worldwide have researched, and are using low-carb, low-fat, high-protein diets to great effect. Recently the 'Total Wellbeing Diet' has gained prominence. Developed by the Commonwealth Scientific and Industrial Research Organisation (CSIRO) in Australia, it recommends high protein and low carbohydrate, with a lower fat intake than Atkins, making it healthier and more balanced. So far, a limited amount of evidence suggests that weight loss occurs simply because of a lower energy intake, assisted by the increased satiety induced by high-protein intake, and that it could be particularly useful in women with metabolic syndrome, especially those with raised triglyceride levels. Diets such as GoLower are now successfully providing low-carbohydrate, high-protein diets, without an increase in fat intake.

The Complete Scarsdale Medical Diet

Dr Herman Tarnower, who practised in Scarsdale, New York, designed his low-carbohydrate, low-energy diet with rigid rules. Published in 1979, its popularity soared after Dr Tarnower was murdered in 1980. That aside, the diet averages 1000 calories a day for females so compliance is poor.

Very-low-fat diets

Following the work of Ansel Keyes in the 1950s, the American Heart Association produced dietary guidelines that promoted a reduction in dietary fat.[6] Keyes had shown that dietary fat consumption, in particular saturated fat, was a strong predictor of coronary heart disease incidence within a population. From this came the Pritikin Diet, essentially focused on reducing heart disease but also contributing to weight loss. However, the Pritikin regimen was difficult to comply with and today has been more or less abandoned, being replaced by other programmes.

Ornish Diet

Currently the best-known very-low-fat diet is that promoted by Dean Ornish, founder and president of the Preventative Medicine Research Institute based in California. The Ornish diet, detailed in the bestseller *Eat More Weigh Less*, recommends a diet containing approximately 10% or less of energy from fat. For this reason, the Ornish diet is extensively and essentially a plant-based or vegetarian diet. There exists a good evidence base for the diet, and researchers have shown in well-conducted clinical trials that compliance with this diet will not only result in weight loss but also in reversal of atherosclerotic plaque.[7]

The diet consists of three food lists: foods that can be eaten all the time, foods that can be eaten in moderation and foods that should be avoided (table 13.1).

The Ornish Diet is based on the principle that when placed on a weight-reducing diet, the human body responds by reducing its basal metabolic rate, thus even eating less food does not result in weight loss. Ornish claims that as his diet represents fewer calories by way of a change, rather than a reduction in food consumption, the effect is different. Therefore the food in the 'permitted' category can be eaten when hungry, dictating that a large number of small meals be eaten each day. In addition, since the diet is high in fibre, there is a slowing of absorption that results in less aggressive stimulation of blood insulin levels and smoother glucose blood concentrations.

Table 13.1 Food types in the Ornish Diet

Foods eaten all the time	Foods eaten in moderation	Foods to be avoided
Beans and legumes	Skimmed milk	Meat
Fruits	Low-fat dairy cheese	Oils, including olive
Grains	Low-fat natural yoghurts	Avocado
Vegetables		Dairy products not low fat

The Ornish Diet promotes a considerable exercise component with a recommendation of a 30-minute session of moderate physical activity every day. In addition the programme recommends stress management techniques such as meditation.

This diet is perhaps the one that is nearest to that currently recommended in government guidelines, although there is an large degree of subjectivity in choosing the appropriate nutritional regime for any given individual.

Some critics suggest that an individual using the Ornish Diet is required to learn a new method of eating – small meals on a regular basis. It is also felt to be very restrictive in the variety of foods that can be eaten, and there is a restriction on certain fats, particularly fish fats, that have been shown to produce heart health, as the regime does not distinguish between 'good' and 'bad' fats.

Glycaemic index diets

Based on the glycaemic index (GI), a ranking system for foods, invented by Dr David Jenkins from the University of Toronto in 1981, the concept is focused on carbohydrates, fruit and vegetables that break down, slowly releasing glucose in the blood stream. A food's glycaemic index is the amount it increases blood glucose levels compared with the amount that same quantity of sugar (which, by definition, has a GI of 100) would increase it. The foods with the lower GI will cause blood glucose to rise and fall more slowly after consumption. Foods with a low GI have been shown in a number of studies to improve satiety, and therefore it is theorised that they reduce appetite and overall energy intake.

In other words, high-GI foods are rapidly absorbed and metabolised, leading to only a transient reduction, followed rapidly by a further carbohydrate craving. Low-GI foods undergo the same process in slow motion, so that they induce an effective 'slow-burn' energy release, avoiding glucose and insulin peaks, and thereby inducing more long-term satiety. The concept of glycaemic load goes one step further, by embracing not just the accessibility of carbohydrates in the diet, but also the amount. For instance, the carbohydrate within a carrot has a similar GI to that within a bar of chocolate, but the chocolate contains far more of it, making it a less suitable snack. Regimes such as Patrick Holford's Glycaemic Load programme take this phenomenon into account, and are therefore potentially more useful. Table 13.2 gives a sample of GI numbers for commonly encountered foods.

Food-combining diets: Hay system

A New Health Era was published by Dr William Hay in the first decade of the 20th century and this diet is still promoted in books such as Food

Table 13.2 Glycaemic index (GI) numbers for common foods

Food	GI	Food	GI
Danish pastry	59	Pears	38
Angel cake	67	Pineapple	66
Orange juice	52	Watermelon	72
Pizza, cheese	60	Baked beans (tin)	48
Wheaten bread	90	Butter beans	31
All-Bran	40	Lentils, green	29
Porridge	49	White spaghetti	41
Weetabix	77	Beetroot	64
Rice Krispies	82	Potato, baked	85
Couscous	65	Potato, boiled	56
Pearl barley	25	Potato, mashed	70
White rice	58	Crisps	54
Digestive biscuits	58	Mars bar	64
Milk, whole	27	Snickers bar	40
Milk, semi-skimmed	34	Tomato soup	38
Ice-cream	61	Honey	58
Low-fat yogurt	33	Liquid glucose	96
Apples	38	French beans	<15
Bananas	54	Tomatoes	15

Combining for Health: A new look at the Hay System by Doris Grant and Jean Joice (1981) and *The Food Combining Diet* by Kathryn Marsden (1993). The Hay System is promoted for weight loss but is also promoted as much for the potential health gains obtained. Dr Hay himself developed poor health and gained excessive weight. Suffering from heart disease, he developed his novel ideas on improved nutrition which had little if any rational scientific basis. He did lose weight, reported and promoted his findings and gathered a lot of followers who also claimed to benefit from the diet. The books and programmes that have revisited the Hay System in recent years claim that Dr Hay has been proved right, as scientific advances provided us with a better understanding of human nutrition and its effect on health – yet these claims are at best spurious.

The Hay System is based on the premise that human diseases have one underlying cause – wrong chemical conditions in the body. Hay claimed that these conditions are created through the manufacture and accumulation of 'acid end-products' of digestion and metabolism in amounts greater than the body can eliminate. This was term 'auto-intoxication, acid-autotoxicosis, toxaemia, self-poisoning . . .'.

Devised in 1911, it is also called the food-combining diet and forbids the combining of 'acid' food with 'alkaline' foods. Acid foods are protein-rich: meat, fish and dairy. Alkaline foods are carbohydrate-rich – rice, grains, potatoes etc.

He claimed that this situation comes about for four reasons:

- by eating too much meat
- over-consumption of refined carbohydrates
- a disregard for the laws of chemistry as they apply to digestion
- constipation.

The Hay System has five rules:

- Starches and sugars should not be eaten with proteins and acid fruits at the same meal.
- Vegetables, salads and fruits should form the major part of the diet.
- Proteins, starches and fats should be eaten in small quantities
- Only whole grain and unprocessed starches should be used and all refined process foods should be ignored.
- An interval of at least 4 hours should elapse between meals of different character.

There is little rationale for this diet; combining foods has no scientific contraindication whatsoever, yet it did induce a reduction in energy intake, and anticipate the problems associated with overconsumption of processed starches, which may explain why the Hay System can effect weight loss in those who use it.

Other diets

Zone Diet

The Zone Diet[10], created by Barry Sears and first published in the US in 1995, focuses on insulin as the key hormone responsible for fat production. Followers of the Zone Diet are encouraged to keep blood insulin levels in a 'tight zone' hence the diet's name. This can be achieved – according to the author – by keeping meals frequent and balanced for fat, carbohydrates and protein. In this way insulin is not stimulated as it might be if the diet contains a large amount of processed carbohydrates, bread, potatoes, pasta etc. In fact, and in common with other diets that focus on insulin, the first 2 weeks on the diet requires total exclusion of carbohydrates, so in this way it is similar to Atkins.

F-Plan Diet

Popularised by Audrey Eyton in the 1970s, and recently reinvigorated, the F-Plan Diet[11] advises consumption of high-fibre foods that were filling without being packed with calories. The diet became identified with baked beans and sales of the staple foods rocketed.

The F-Plan Diet is based on an increase in dietary fibre that encourages satiety at a lower level of energy intake and, to a lesser extent, by increasing the amount of potential energy lost in the faeces. This was endorsed by the Royal College of Physicians in their early reports on obesity that further added to the popularity of the diet in the 1980s. Less sugar and fat are, crucially, key elements of a healthy diet.

In the 1970s, when the F-Plan Diet was introduced, there had been a steady decline in the fibre content in the Western diet. Food processing stripped the fibre out of food to make it more palatable, although a lack of dietary fibre is now linked to bowel cancer and heart disease. A diet that promotes a higher consumption of whole cereal foods, fruit and vegetables is clearly in line with good nutritional guidelines. The F-Plan Diet programme increased consumption of dietary fibre to between 30 and 50 g per day.

Certainly those who follow the F-Plan Diet do experience greater satiety from the high-fibre food recommended. A small study reported by Geoffery Cannon in *Dieting Makes You Fat* showed that those who ate wholemeal bread (lightly buttered) to satiety only consumed 665 kcal, compared with those who ate white bread to satiety, when this group had consumed 825 kcal. The effect is similar to Dr Burkitt's 'Irish Diet' (see above).

Jumping on the F-Plan Diet's success has meant that many foods identified with the diet may not be as healthy as assumed. For example, baked beans, a key element of the F-Plan Diet, contain 5% processed sugar, and some of the breakfast cereal can contain up to 15% processed sugar.

Rosemary Conley's Hip and Thigh Diet

Rosemary Conley's Hip and Thigh Diet[12] was an international bestseller in the 1990s, based on a low-fat regimen combined with exercise in the form of an aerobic workout.

The No-Diet Diet

Ben Fletcher and colleagues, with a background in human psychology, have developed a unique weight-loss programme paradoxically called the No-Diet

Diet (NDD). As a weight-loss intervention it at first appears counterintuitive, since it claims to have nothing to do with food directly; rather the programme attempts to empower the individual to take greater personal control of his or her decision making. In this way, it is argued, people lose weight because they do things differently. The No-Diet Diet is based on an idea that each individual's behaviour is controlled by a series of habits or pre-programmed responses. Perhaps 85% of our daily actions (behaviours) are controlled in this way and because of this, bad habits are ingrained and make any form of change difficult. The authors define a 'habitweb' for each individual in which the source of being overweight is centred.

With some scientific evidence to support this idea, the NDD is founded in the Framework of Internal Transformation (FIT) a tool for measuring an individual's psychology and a means of effecting change. FIT identifies five areas of thinking – the 'inner FIT elements' – termed constancies (box 13.2), and 15 areas of behaviour – the 'outer FIT elements'. These include assertive/unassertive, reactive/proactive, definite/flexible, risky/cautious.

The authors of the diet argue that a combination of these 'inner' and 'outer' FIT elements determines how a person sees him or herself and more importantly behaves in the way that they do. From the FIT framework, the authors offer a means of change that will allow the individual to break ingrained habits and in this way dismantle their personal 'habitweb' – the linking of habits that lead to being overweight or obese.

'By changing the things we do, we have a lever for changing the way we view the world by an alteration in our way of thinking.'

This, according to the diet's designers, allows individuals to gain better control of ingrained habits and in turn this allows them to more easily achieve goals such as losing weight. Through behavioural flexibility, individuals are able to:

- change behaviour whenever required
- act after a conscious decision rather than from just habit
- try new ways of dealing with situations
- allow others to do things their own way.

Box 13.2 The five constancies (inner FIT elements)

- self-responsibility
- awareness
- conscience
- fearlessness
- balance

The programme agrees that employing a simple energy-restrictive diet fails to address core behaviours that have resulted in the individual being over-weight in the first place. The authors cite poor eating, and exercise habits that are locked in a negative spiral. For example, watching television is often linked to resting, eating and drinking. Habits have numerous links and often habits that have a bearing on what and how much we eat may be distant from dietary habits. Dieters often fail to lose weight in the long-term since dietary habits are tackled in isolation of the linked habits. By increasing behavioural flexibility – doing things differently – the programme attempts to support sustainable weight loss without requiring compliance with complex nutritional or exercise programmes.

To be effective in both weight loss and in reducing disease risk, the NDD requires a understanding of healthy nutrition. With additional research it might prove a major advance in weight management in the long term and is a concept that could be easily incorporated into a pharmacy-based obesity programme to support the behaviour element.

How do the diets stack up?

A systematic review and meta-analysis of the literature surrounding the different regimes, involving people who completed weight loss clinical trials on diet alone, diet and exercise and meal replacements resulted in a mean weight loss of 5–8 kg (5–9% over 6 months). Weight loss plateaued at 6 months and stabilised at a weight loss of approximately 4.5–7 kg (4.8%–8.0%) at 12 months. Weight loss was maintained at 24, 36 and 48 months at about 3–4 kg (3–4.3%) with none of the groups experiencing weight gain to baseline.

Very-low-energy diets can result in dramatic weight loss, but may also be followed by rapid and substantial weight gain, unless long-term behav-ioural techniques are adopted.

Exercise alone or advice alone, even when accompanied by written infor-mation or individual one-to-one sessions, did not result in successful weight loss, although no further weight gain was observed in these two types of interventions. Patients must continue with a lower energy diet and regular physical activity to prevent weight regain and this is often difficult, and a key factor in the lack of long-term efficacy of a weight-loss programme.

Findings from the US National Weight Control registry[6] suggest that people who are most successful in maintaining weight that they have lost, do three things;

- They eat breakfast
- They have regular physical activity (30 to 60 minutes per day).
- They weigh themselves once a week

Diet quality

The quality of a range of weight-reduction diets was assessed using the alternate healthy eating index (AHEI), a measure that isolates dietary components most strongly linked to cardiovascular risk reduction. Factors included in this index include: fruit and vegetables, nuts, ratio of white to red meat, cereal fibre, ratio of polyunsaturated fat to trans fats.

Not surprisingly, none of the popular commercial diets achieved a perfect AHEI score. However, the Ornish Diet, owing to its vegetarian element, achieved the highest score, as would be expected due to the quantities of fruit, vegetables and cereal fibre and avoidance of trans fats. The Weight Watchers Higher Carbohydrate Diet and the New Glucose Revolution did well, again because of their emphasis on fruit and vegetables, wholegrain and low trans fats.

The Atkins diet had the lowest score, mainly because of the lack of fruit and vegetables and non-starch polysaccharides, although it did result in the greatest intake of omega-3-fatty acids; however, saturated fat was high, ranging from 16.2% to 17.6% of total energy intake. Those diets that conformed to the recommendations of less than 10% of saturated fat of total energy included Weight Watchers, the New Glucose Revolution, Ornish and the Zone Diet.

Dr Atkins and similar diets such as Lipotrim increase blood ketones. High-blood ketones are associated with feelings of fatigue and mood disturbances while exercising, suggesting that low-carbohydrate diets could reduce the desire to exercise; this would be counterproductive in people attempting to lose weight.

In the only long-term study[13] on the effects of low-carbohydrate diets, there was no evidence of an increased risk of coronary heart disease. This study involved tracking 82 800 women over a 20-year period. It should be remembered that heart disease rates are higher in men. The reason for this finding was that there seemed to be no difference in the risk of coronary heart disease between high-fat and high-carbohydrate diets. This might be explained by the fact that vegetable fat is associated with a lower risk of disease, whereas high-carbohydrate diets involving large quantities of high-GI carbohydrates that can rapidly elevate blood sugar, were associated with increased risk of coronary heart disease.

A second study over a 5-year period[14] compared the effect of low-carbohydrate, high-protein diets on overall mortality in 22 944 adult men and women. The findings were that a high intake of protein was associated with a slight increase in total mortality while a high-carbohydrate diet was associated with a reduction in total mortality. A diet low in carbohydrate and high in protein was associated with a 22% (significant) increase in overall mortality.

A Swedish study that followed 42 000 women for 12 years[15] found that a low-carbohydrate, high protein diet was associated with increased mortality, particularly coronary heart disease.

Conclusion

High-carbohydrate diets used in the management of weight control do reduce BMI. Evidence from a review demonstrated that avoiding carbohydrates with a high GI helps to prevent conditions such as cardiovascular disease, type 2 diabetes or cancer, from which it was concluded that a low-carbohydrate, low-fat diet is still best.[16]

Clearly the most effective diet to reduce weight is one that is a minimum of 500 kcal (600 kcal would be better) deficient per day less than a person's requirement. This should be coupled with moderate exercise daily, 30 minutes minimum, preferably 60 minutes. A high-carbohydrate but low-GI diet is preferable. The healthiest type of carbohydrate is still unclear but there is some evidence that a low-GI diet helps to improve fullness and increase weight loss. This will be particularly true in people with hyper-insulinaemia, diabetes and metabolic syndrome.[16]

The Cochrane database assessed randomised, controlled trials that compared weight loss in people eating higher GI diets and found that people eating low-GI foods lost significantly more weight than those on other diets.[17]

A small study in 30 schoolchildren aged 8–11 years found that children who ate a low-GI breakfast consumed an average of 60 calories less than those who ate a high-GI breakfast.[18]

References

1. Cannon G, Einzig H. *Dieting Makes You Fat: a guide to energy, food, fitness and health*. London: Sphere, 1984.
2. Atkins R. *Dr Atkin's New Diet Revolution*. London: Random House, 1992.
3. Costain L. *Diet Trials: how to succeed at dieting*. London: BBC, 2003.
4. Agatston A. *The South Beach Diet: the doctor's plan for fast and lasting weight loss*. London: Headline, 2003.
5. Clark C. *The New High Protein Diet*. London: Vermillion, 2004.
6. Lichienstein A. Very low fat diets. *Circulation* 1998; 98: 935–939.
7. Stephenson J. Low-carb, low fat diet gurus face off. *JAMA* 2003; 289: 1767–1773.
8. Mason P. Weight loss update. *Independent Community Pharmacy*, Nov 2007: 28–30.
9. Halton T L *et al*. Low-carbohydrate-diet score and the risk of coronary heart disease in women. *New Engl J Med* 2006; 355: 1991–2002.
10. Sears B. *The Zone Diet*. London: Thorsons (HarperCollins), 1999.
11. Eyton A. *Audrey Eyton's Extraordinary F-Plan Diet*. London: Penguin, 1982.
12. Conley R. *Rosemary Conley's Complete Hip and Thigh Diet*. London: Arrow, 1989.
13. Gaesser G A. Carbohydrate quantity and quality in relation to body mass index. *J Am Diet Assoc* 2007; 107; 1768–1780.

14. Trichopoulou A *et al.* Low-carbohydrate-high-protein diet and long-term survival in a general population cohort. *Eur J Clin Nutr* 2007; 61: 575–581.

15. Lagiou P *et al.* Low carbohydrate-high protein diet and mortality in a cohort of Swedish women. *J Intern Med* 2007; 261: 366–374.

16. McMullan-Price J *et al.* Comparison of 4 diets of varying glycemic load on weight loss and cardiovascular risk reduction in overweight and obese young adults: a randomized controlled trial. *Arch Intern Med* 2006; 166: 1466–1475.

17. Thomas D E *et al.* Low glycaemic index or low glycaemic load diets for overweight and obesity. *Cochrane Database Sys Rev* 2007 Jul 18(3); CD005105.

18. Henry C J *et al.* Effects of long-term intervention with low- and high-glycaemic-index breakfasts on food intake in children aged 8–11 years. *Br J Nutr* 2007; 98: 636–640.

14

Over-the-counter slimming aids

For many people, exercise and a reduced-energy diet, coupled with the need for constant avoidance of tempting, tasty energy-rich foods just seems too difficult. Over-the-counter (OTC) dietary slimming aids, available without a prescription, that promise easy weight loss are clearly an attractive proposition.

Historical background

Supposed weight-reduction agents have been available directly to the public for many years and had their hey-day in the Victorian era, when robust evidence for a product was neither offered nor sought, regulation was non-existent, and postal and newspaper advertising was suddenly overwhelmingly powerful. With no genuine weight-loss products available, the market was suddenly wide open for companies or individuals to hawk and peddle their wares to a gullible population. Cancer cures were popular, remedies for tiredness, nervous disorders and men and women's 'weaknesses' sold well, and obesity cures were among the bestsellers, and most profitable.

One of the first remedies of the 'New Era', in 1893, was the 'unexcelled blood-purifier', Allan's AntiFat, a harmless, vegetable-based remedy sold at many stockists. As is standard for preparations lacking evidence of efficacy, preparations relied on unvalidated testimonials. Allan's AntiFat caused 'a lady' to reduce by 25 pounds (11 kg), and she exclaimed 'I hope to never regain what I have lost'. The American Medical Association analysed the product, and discovered the presence of toxic compounds, including mercury, strychnine, arsenic and even tobacco. But the risk of toxicity from such preparations was not a priority for the consumer, and even tapeworms have allegedly been bought and sold for their weight-reducing effect. Although the precise compounds, and the advertising media have changed, the cynical sentiments behind the flogging of useless anti-obesity products to a gullible public are still thriving.

Lack of evidence

With compliance to conventional weight management programmes notoriously poor, there is a case for safe, effective and acceptable therapeutic options and with a greater emphasis currently on self-care, this becomes a higher priority in societies where obesity is a major public health problem. Certainly OTC slimming-aid products are already widely available and have been for many years. Pharmacy shelves stock sensible, scientifically validated weight-loss remedies, such as meal replacement therapies, and low-energy diets, which are effective, and deemed appropriate by NICE and other bodies, but also contain other, more questionable compounds, which are aggressively marketed to the public but whose actual efficacy in contrast to the claims on the pack, remains an issue. Many of these products are not pharmaceutical agents, therefore pharmacists, doctors, other healthcare professionals and even obesity specialists know little about them, yet their usage is widespread. In a recent survey of 460 pharmacy customers, 20% claimed to have tried an OTC weight-loss product. Some 60% thought that an assessment of weight and height should be taken before supply of these products is made.[1]

Manufacturers of OTC slimming aids claim that their products induce significant weight loss without unwanted side-effects, yet many of their ingredients have never undergone rigorous scientific testing and claims about effectiveness are often at best misleading. Unless a product is a licensed medicine as in the case of Alli (OTC orlistat 60-mg capsules) then it is unlikely that the consumer will achieve any weight loss enhanced by the product, and will be subjected to potential adverse events.

Recently in the UK, the Advertising Standards Agency (ASA) instructed the manufactures of 'Pink Patch' to take down their website targeted specifically at young women. The claims they made for the Pink Patch on the website were, according to a ruling by the ASA, unsubstantiated and the amount of product that needed to be purchased were viewed to be excessive.

The Pink Patch is a good example of the type of product designed solely to be sold as an OTC aid to weight loss but for which there is no evidence, either for the effectiveness of the actual ingredients, or that the technology – a pharmaceutical patch – works in delivering the ingredients into the body. Instructions for use are that one patch is applied to the skin daily. The makers claim the formulation contains *Fucus vesiculosus* (bladder wrack), 5-hydroxytryptophan, guarana, zinc pyruvate, yerba mate, flaxseed oil, lecithin and L-carnitine.

The company behind the agent claim that the manufacturing process for the Pink Patch complies with FDA Good Manufacturing Practice (GMP) yet with no FDA approval for the product, either as a food or as a medicine, the validity of this claim cannot be easily investigated. Verification of compliance with GMP will only be provided on product licensing and batch approval. There is no means of knowing what amount (concentration) of each 'active' ingredient is contained in each patch. This product is not licensed and therefore not subject to inspection by government agencies.

Furthermore, there is no way of discovering, in the absence of proper licensing information, if the 'active' ingredients in each patch are able or capable of crossing the skin barrier and therefore entering the blood system. Only by transferring across the skin could the product be effective. Few natural products readily cross the skin, which acts as a natural barrier to keep products out of the body. Patch formulations require chemical modification of drugs to ensure their efficient transcutaneous passage is achieved. Pharmaceutical assessment does not appear to have been undertaken for this product, and would need to be done for each of the 'active' ingredients and is a costly and time-consuming process.

The various ingredients claimed to exist in the Pink Patch have had an association with the OTC slimming industry for many years, despite misgivings about their efficacy (see below). it seems that current policy is to clump as many of these ingredients together to convince consumers that where one ingredient is good, more is better. The Pink Patch had a precursor that was based on bladder wrack (*F. vesiculosus*), a naturally occurring seaweed and recognised source of iodine. Fucus was taken by fat Victorians to assist weight loss, at the same time as Irish farmers were using it to fatten pigs. In a patch widely marketed in the 1980s, 'Le Patch', the manufacturer claimed that this source of iodine was sufficient to improve thyroid function. Low thyroid function is associated with weight gain but iodine supplementation would only be effective where a genuine deficiency in iodine existed, a rare if not non-existent condition in developed countries. Thyroid dysfunction can be a serious medical condition and must be referred for medical assessment.

Marketing genius

What manufacturers of most OTC slimming-aid products lack in basic pharmaceutical science and pharmacology, they make up for in marketing excellence. They are masters of the four Ps of marketing: product, price, place and promotion, from which they create the product's marketing mix. Marketing is so successful that some of these products achieve multi-million pound annual sales.

The product – the OTC slimming aid – is generally formulated to look like a medicine: a capsule, a tablet or a patch, giving the impression to the consumer of a medically effective product. Products are expensive, therefore desirable. Marketing theory suggests that if someone purchases a product that is expensive he or she is more likely, not wishing to lose face, to convince himself of the product's curative properties, even when there is none. Placement of the product is mostly in pharmacies and in herbal shops. The placement in pharmacies is an important part of the marketing mix, as the product's reputation benefits from its association with the pharmacist's. For this reason, pharmacists in particular must carefully consider the implications of stocking and selling such products. A discussion of the ethical consideration appeared in the *Pharmaceutical Journal* in 2008[2] in which the author suggested that: 'There is clearly a need for a look at how the OTC slimming aid market is being regulated since current regulation is failing to protect the public and perhaps is acting against public health. That said there is also a need for community pharmacies to be more circumspect with a product that make significant claims about losing weight'.

Will community pharmacy continue to supply products of questionable quality and efficacy? Probably, but if they do they run the risk of damaging their considerable reputation. We must keep standards high and only sell things we can stand by. To do anything else is as ridiculous as a religious bookshop selling soft porn.

Promotion, the last of the four Ps, is where manufacturers are at their most inventive. In most countries, strict regulations control product claims, particularly those relating to health. Manufacturers have been highly inventive and creative in overcoming these restrictions, and as a result, in getting their message across. Whereas medical claims for foods and medicines are not allowed, some manufacturers have found ways around this restriction. Traditionally, this was done using personal testimonies used to convince others, for example: 'I could never lose weight until I tried Brand X, now I am a size 10 for the first time in my life.' Yet some manufacturers have been even more inventive and have found a way of manipulating the product regulatory system.

Formoline LU11, a German slimming product registered as a medical device within the EU and launched in the UK in 2008, claims to reduce energy intake from dietary fats, assist long-term weight control and lower low-density lipoprotein cholesterol. If the product were a food or a medicine, it would be illegal to make such claims. However, these claims are made on the basis of the product being registered as a medical device.

The Advertising Standards Authority (ASA) upheld a series of complaints about claims made for a similar product called LIPObind. When queried by the ASA, the Medicines and Healthcare Products Regulatory Authority (MHRA) accepted the fat-binding and weight management claims for LIPObind on the grounds that its performance was assessed by a 'Notified Body'. A Notified Body is any group that are capable of assessing the claims and submitting evidence to the regulatory authority. On following up the evidence, ASA found that the claims could not be backed up by rigorous scientific trails in people. These products contain chitosan or chitosan-like polymers.

OTC diet-aid products

There exist on the market a huge and complex variety of OTC weight control products. The ingredients of these products are thought to act by either one or all of the following mechanisms:

- increase satiety
- decrease in absorption
- increase fat oxidation, increase metabolic rate, or reduce lipogenesis.

Examples of some of these ingredients include L-carnitine and acetyl-L-carnitine, chitosan, chromium, fibre, hydroxycitric acid (HCA), seaweed, green tea, conjugated linoleic acid and lecithin.

With the exception of Alli, which is available OTC in the US and Europe, and for which there is good evidence of safety and efficacy, there is little evidence that other OTC slimming aids work. What follows is an assessment of the current published evidence for the efficacy and safety of the ingredients of popular OTC slimming products. This assessment is based on four detailed review articles.[3–6]

Ephedra sinica

Historically, sympathomimetic amines have been used as over-the-counter diet aids, including phenylpropanolamine, *ma huang* (ephedra) and ephedrine. A systematic review of five double-blinded trials concluded that the combination of ephedrine and caffeine is effective in reducing body weight. The most rigorous review[7], which assessed human studies for longer than 8 weeks, concluded that *E. sinica* and ephedrine promote a modest short-term weight loss of approximately 0.9 kg per month greater than placebo.

It is effective but this efficacy has been associated with a threefold increase in side-effects including psychiatric events, gastrointestinal events and heart palpitations. Indeed, these products became notorious for causing dose-related increases in blood pressure, which may not be problematic in healthy patients but can be hazardous in others. When the use of phenylpropanolamine was correlated with hypertension and stroke, the FDA banned it from the US market in 2000. Likewise, *ma huang* and ephedrine-containing supplements have been removed from the US market.

There currently exist few OTC products with the potential to improve thermogenic properties yet where this is suggested in product promotional material, overweight patients often are willing to give these new products a try, even in the absence of properly conducted clinical trials.

Chitosan

Products that contain chitosan include:

- Fat Magnets
- LipoBind capsules (chitosan-like polymer)
- Liposorb capsules
- Strobby tablets
- Fat Binder
- Bonsal

Chitosan, is a cationic polysaccharide, and is a derivative of a chitin found in shells of invertebrates, such as crabs and shrimp. It has a highly adsorptive surface and for this reason is widely promoted as a 'fat blocker.' Animal studies have shown that chitosan can reduce body weight and a small number of studies in humans have shown a similar effect but many suffer from poor methodology and therefore provide a poor evidence base for chitosan-based products.

A meta-analysis has identified five studies evaluating the effectiveness of chitosan in obesity management.[8] Mean weight loss with chitosan was 3.3 kg, greater than placebo but major methodological flaws in the studies were identified which greatly limits the conclusion. A well-performed double-blind trial found no significant differences in BMI in 30 overweight individuals receiving chitosan and placebo, yet this has not been repeated in other studies and there is evidence to suggest that the proposed mechanism by which chitosan effects weight loss – fat retention in the gut and expulsion in faeces – does not work. In one study, 7 healthy males consumed >120 g fat per day for 12 days and took chitosan prior to meals and snacks on days 6–9 (15 capsules or 5.25 g chitosan per day). Faecal samples were collected on days 2–12 and were analysed for fat content. Fat content of the faeces did not change from the chitosan-free period, and the authors concluded that the chitosan did not block fat absorption.[9]

In another study, 250 patients were randomised in a 24-week, double-blind, placebo-controlled trial to receive 3 g chitosan per day or placebo. Chitosan treatment did not result in a clinically significant loss of body weight or a significant difference in adverse events.[9]

Other scientific studies confirm these findings[5] and therefore the evidence available in the literature indicates that there is considerable doubt that chitosan is effective for reducing body weight in humans. Adverse events most frequently included gastrointestinal symptoms such as constipation and flatulence.

Hoodia gordanii

Trim Easy is claimed to work as an appetite suppressant. Manufacturers of products containing hoodia claim it to be the first truly effective weight management product. Hoodia is derived from the cactus *Hoodia gordanii*, which grows in the Kalahari Desert. Manufacturers claim that, for thousands of years, the bushmen of South Africa have used hoodia to stave off hunger during hunting trips that might last weeks. Featured in a BBC television programme, *60 Minutes*, in 2004 the BBC endorsed the manufacturers' claims and the fact that the plant extract was without side-effects. An active ingredient, P57, was isolated by the company Phytopharm who claim to have undertaken double-blind, placebo-controlled clinical studies in overweight, but otherwise healthy volunteers using the extract.[10]

The participants were split into two groups, one group received the P57 and the other received a placebo. Both groups were told to continue their normal diet and exercise. The results, unpublished in a peer-reviewed scientific journal, suggested that the P57 group had a significant reduction in body fat associated with a reduction in daily energy intake compared with placebo but with no side-effects. Indeed Phytopharm claimed that the P57 group ate about 1000 fewer kilocalories per day, speculating that hoodia, or more specifically P57 extract, imitates the effect of glucose on brain neurones. There is little to support this claim or indeed objective evidence of efficacy but Phytopharm made a serious attempt to isolate and endorse a product that, if it proves to work, would have a huge commercial value and might even make a considerable contribution to public health.

Phytopharm theorised that following a meal, blood sugar levels rise and trigger a satiety centre in the brain that stops eating. P57 is claimed to mimic an endogenous satiety neuroligand. Hoodia products, in common with most OTC weight control products, are licensed as food supplements and therefore product quality does not require the rigour required for a licensed medicine. Phytopharm used this as a key marketing ploy, suggesting inferiority of their competitor's product. Development of P57 stalled, and the product has since been passed between pharmaceutical giants, without seeing the light of day. However, it is still described as a 'pipeline product', and may yet prove to be a genuine weight loss agent in the future.

Chromium picolinate

Products that contain chromium include:

- Fat Blaster
- LipoBind.

Chromium is an essential trace element involved in carbohydrate and fat metabolism. Since chromium can enhance insulin sensitivity, decrease circulating insulin levels and improve glucose tolerance, it has been theorised that it could increase satiety, improve body composition (ratio of lean to fat tissue), increase basal metabolic rate and reduce body weight. There currently is no evidence base to support this, with most studies being poor and few reporting efficacy.

Chromium picolinate is an organic compound, which is the main presentation for chromium in OTC slimming products. A meta-analysis of 10 double-blinded RCTs suggested a relatively small reduction of 1.1–1.2 kg compared with placebo in interventions that lasted 6–14 weeks and that this weight loss was not significantly meaningful.

Oral chromium is relatively non-toxic but there are reports of excessive doses of chromium being associated with renal impairment and rhabomyolysis (muscle wasting due to muscle cell death).

L-Carnitine and acetyl-L-carnitine

L-Carnitine is a cofactor in cellular fat oxidation, which is diminished in obesity because of a reduction in L-carnitine enzyme-related activity. For this theoretical reason, L-carnitine is promoted as a 'fat-burner', despite little if any evidence to support its efficacy in obese or overweight humans. In a study on rodents, it was found that compared with placebo, a diet supplemented with L-carnitine was no better at inducing weight loss compared with an energy-restricted diet. A study looking at basketball players, a group that was lean before the study began, showed a reduction in body fat associated with L-carnitine use but not in overall body mass.[11] Overall there is little evidence to support the clinical efficacy of this product, as no properly controlled clinical trials have demonstrated its effectiveness in weight loss.

Acetyl-L-carnitine is metabolically similar to L-carnitine and *in vitro* is capable of restoring mitochondrial energy production, and thus is claimed by some to increase energy expenditure. Although some small studies in rodents have shown weight loss associated with acetyl-L-carnitine supplementation, there has been no scientific evidence for weight loss in humans.[4]

Green tea

Green tea has been promoted as a weight-loss supplement for over 20 years and in recent times there has been renewed interest in its use. Green tea contains catechin polyphenols, which have been shown to inhibit COMT, the enzyme responsible for the degradation of noradrenaline. Since noradrenaline has an important role in the control of thermogenesis, basal metabolic rate and fat metabolism, it has been theorised that consumption of green tea might contribute to weight loss. Work in rats has demonstrated weight loss but this is restored once supplementation is stopped. Tea catechin has been shown to cause appetite loss, which might be the route by which the weight loss is effected.

A small study in humans (n = 10) has shown that green tea increased 24-hour energy expenditure.[12] Interestingly, in this study that compared green tea, caffeine and placebo, caffeine was shown to have no effect on energy expenditure. However, a larger study over a longer period of time looked at the weight gain in a group who had lost 7.5% of body weight through dieting. Green tea was no better than placebo in halting the regain of weight and there was no noted increase in metabolism in the green-tea group. Green tea is relatively safe given the number of people who routinely use it as a daily beverage, and no side-effects were reported in these studies.

Conjugated linoleic acid

Studies in rodents have demonstrated a reduction in body fat and body weight after treatment with conjugated linoleic acid (CLA) supplements. For this reason CLA supplements have been promoted OTC as a weight-loss aid. However, there is little evidence that CLA supplements reduce body weight or body fat in humans. More worryingly, studies in rodents have shown that CLA supplementation is associated with liver hypertrophy and insulin resistance and this must be of concern to anyone wishing to use them. However no human trials to date have demonstrated such adverse events, even in higher than normal doses.[4]

CLA is thought to achieve its weight loss effect in rodents by a number of routes: increased energy expenditure, reduced fat cell size, increasing apoptosis of fat cells and the inhibition of lipogenesis in the liver or increasing fat oxidation. For this reason and since CLA is a complex mixture of linoleic acids bonded at different locations, it might be that not all CLA supplement are equivalent. One clinical trial, which suggested that there was little evidence of efficacy, concentrated only on studies that incorporated *trans*-10 and *cis*-12 isomers. About 90% of CLA from food intake is in the form of *cis*-9 and *trans*-11 isomers. A lack of standardisation of CLA isomers in studies may explain the often contradictory evidence from scientific studies.

Hydroxycitric acid

Products that contain hydroxycitric acid include:

- Fat Blaster
- Healthtrim tablets.

Hydroxycitric acid is obtained from extracts of *Garcinia cambogia* and has been shown to inhibit the citrate cleavage enzyme, suppress *de-novo* fatty acid synthesis and food intake. In this way it is theorised it decreases body weight gain.

Although a number of studies in humans support the efficacy of HCA in weight loss, all studies suffer from significant methodological deficiencies that bring the relevance of the findings into question. For example, in some studies HCA was administered in combination with chromium or chitosan or used with a low-fat diet, making an assessment of the effect of HCA difficult. In one study two groups were assessed, one on a low-energy diet and the other on the same low-energy diet with HCA supplementation. Both groups were followed over 12 weeks and, although both groups lost significant amounts of weight, there was no difference between them.[13]

In one double-blind, randomised, controlled trial, which tested the benefits of 3 g *G. cambogia* extract in patients with an average BMI of 32 kg/m^2, results suggested the absence of a significantly greater weight loss in the treatment group than in the placebo group[6] yet other studies show conflicting results. Overall the evidence is not compelling and adverse events have been reported and include headache, upper respiratory tract symptoms and gastrointestinal symptoms, particularly stomach pain.

Non-starch polysaccharides (fibre)

Products that contain fibre include:

- Fibre Slim
- Vitafibre
- Celluvac.

Based on the F-Plan Diet theme, some commercial companies identified an opportunity to market fibre-based products that increase satiety and so reduce energy intake. Where this has been shown to happen, for example, in the context of the F-Plan Diet, the amount of fibre needed to support and maintain weight loss is larger than the amount normally provided from fibre supplements. There exists no evidence that these supplements can induce significant weight loss in the long term.[4]

Certainly a high consumption of fibre supplements is associated with bloating, diarrhoea and nausea. Large quantities of bran may reduce absorption of vitamins and minerals – not a problem with water-soluble fibres (pectin and psyllium).

Herbal diuretics

Products that contain herbal diuretics include:

- Adios (boldo and dandelion root)
- Waterban.

Diuretics, both herbal and pharmaceutical, have been widely used for weight loss. Sportsmen, such as Olympic wrestlers sometimes took them before a match, in order to make the correct weight for the bout. Although weight is temporarily reduced, due to the reduction in fluid load, there are no health benefits conferred by these products, except when correctly prescribed for separate conditions. Dandelion has long been known to have diuretic effect, and laxative properties; Culpeper referred to dandelion as 'piss-a-beds': 'It openeth the passages of the urine both in young and old; powerfully cleanseth imposthumes and inward ulcers in the urinary passages ... And whoever is drawing towards a consumption, or an evil disposition of the whole body ... shall find a wonderful help. It helpeth also to procure rest and sleep to bodies distempered by the heat of ague-fits, or otherwise.'

There seems to be no evidence of modern usage of these products, and the situation is unlikely to change, given the spurious and transient nature of any weight loss induced.

Lecithin

Products that contain lecithin include:

- Nature's Aid Trim-it.

Lecithin is a phospholipid found in egg yolks, liver, peanuts and soya beans. Lecithin is thought to prevent the deposition of fat in fat cells. A well-conducted Swedish study examining the effect of lecithin supplementation and its effect on weight did not find any significant benefits in weight loss.

Guarana and yerba mate

Yerba mate (*Ilex paraguariensis*) is an evergreen tree that is native to South America. It is often combined in OTC weight-loss preparation with guarana (*Paullinia cupana*).

Both these plants are sources of stimulant chemical agents, caffeine and xanthine, respectively. There is some evidence that extracts from these plants that are very high in caffeine have been able to prolong gastric emptying time. However, there is little evidence that, as stimulants, they are effective in raising the body's basal metabolic rate to such a degree as to cause weight loss. There is, however, evidence that pseudoephedrine (a related chemical stimulant) is effective in doing this and there have been some cases where 'natural' slimming aids containing these plant extracts were adulterated with pseudoephedrine and this has been associated with adverse events on the heart.[3]

5-Hydroxytryptophan

Hydroxytrytophan (5-HTP) is a naturally occurring amino acid that is thought to have a mild psychoactive effect. It can cross the blood-brain barrier and in the brain is metabolised to 5-HT (serotonin), a brain neurotransmitter associated with depression when deficient. 5-HTP is normally sold as a food supplement in doses of 50–100 mg per tablet for oral use. There is some evidence of its efficacy in treating depression but not for its role in weight control. Serotonin, noradrenaline and dopamine are all neurotransmitters associated with both mood and appetite regulation. The modern generation of prescribable antidepressants – selective serotonin reuptake inhibitors (SSRIs) – act by increasing serotonin, and sometimes noradrenaline levels in the brain. The SSRI fluoxetine (Prozac) was noted to induce mild weight loss during the first 6 months of treatment, and sibutramine, a similar compound, was found to have no effect on mood, but to induce significant weight loss, and is now successfully marketed as a weight-loss drug. These prescription products are clearly not available over the counter.

Plantago psyllium

Psyllium is a water-soluble fibre derived from the husks of ripe seeds of *Plantago ovata*. One double-blind randomised, controlled trial, which included patients with type 2 diabetes and a mean BMI of 29 kg/m^2, found no significant changes in body weight in either the treatment or the placebo group. There were no reports of side-effects.

Hydroxmethylbutyrate

Hydroxmethylbutyrate is a metabolite of leucine that has been shown to have anti-catabolic action through inhibiting protein breakdown. Products containing HMB are primarily targeted at body builders who wish to change body composition and improve muscle mass. There is some evidence to support this outcome but the few trials that are published have methodological problems and therefore more studies are required.

Pyruvate

Pyruvate is created in the body through glycolysis. Supplementation with pyruvate seems to enhance exercise performance and improve measures of body composition. There exist two randomised, controlled trials involving patients with a BMI of 25 kg/m² or more but neither showed any greater effect on weight compared with placebo so the conclusion is that pyruvate is an aid to body composition changes but that weight loss is weak.

Orlistat

Orlistat (Alli) is the only FDA-approved over-the-counter medication currently approved for weight loss. It was launched in the US in 2007 and in many European countries following EMEA approval in April 2009. The drug selectively inhibits gastrointestinal and pancreatic lipase activity, resulting in a 25–33% reduction of dietary fat absorption.

Orlistat has been available by prescription in a dose of 120 mg (Xenical), where the evidence for its use is robust, and was switched to OTC firstly in the US where the FDA approved a 60-mg dose 3 times daily with meals or shortly after. A reduced-calorie diet, smaller meal portions, and a maximum of 15 g of fat per meal are recommended by the manufacturer. Side-effects are minimal, with most common adverse events being gastrointestinal, most often caused by more fat consumption than is recommended.

The pivotal studies from the original orlistat 120 mg licence were supportive for orlistat 60 mg, the OTC strength. These studies were double-blind, double-dummy, randomised, parallel-group, placebo-controlled, multicentre studies and included a 60-mg arm as well as the 120-mg arm. The main objective of these studies was to determine the weight-loss effect of 60 mg orlistat, 120 mg orlistat, or placebo administered three times daily in combination with a mildly hypocaloric diet, during the first year of treatment.[14]

One study, a multicentre, double-blind, randomised, placebo-controlled, parallel-group study conducted in overweight patients with a BMI of 25 kg/m² or more and under 28 kg/m² assessed the efficacy of orlistat 60 mg three times daily plus diet compared with placebo plus diet on change in the body weight over 16 weeks in subjects with BMI of 25 kg/m² or more to under 28 kg/m².[15]

Orlistat 60 mg was shown to increase weight loss in overweight and obese subjects compared with placebo. The weight loss increases with increased baseline BMI measurements such that the obese subject benefited more than the overweight or normal weight subject.

Results demonstrate efficacy of the 60 mg strength in subjects with a BMI of 28 kg/m² or more with 45% achieving a weight loss of over 5% of baseline body weight and 21% achieving a weight loss of over 10% of baseline body weight (compared with 29.3% and 11.5% respectively in the placebo group). This degree of weight loss is clinically significant with regard to the risk factors for diabetes and cardiovascular disease.

There was less evidence of efficacy in subjects with a BMI of 25–28 kg/m^2 and the OTC licence indication will be for individuals with a BMI of 28 kg/m^2 or more. In these subjects the actual weight loss was small (3–4.5 kg over 3–4 months) and only 1.15 kg more than the placebo group on average but appears to continue while the medication is taken and not to plateau after a short time.

In further studies, results for the 60 mg dose remained significant in all the sensitivity analyses at 6 months but the baseline carried forward analysis was not significant for the 60 mg dose at 12 months.

Whereas the effect size is modest and smaller than seen with the prescription-only approved dose of 120 mg, its clinical relevance could be associated with a significant public health gain.

Withdrawal

Two studies conducted with orlistat 120 mg demonstrated some weight gain following discontinuation of therapy. However these patients were allowed to take a eucaloric diet rather than being encouraged to continue a low-energy diet. Importantly the results did not demonstrate a 'rebound' weight gain where the weight rose to above the baseline weight. The success of any attempt to lose weight is dependent upon the consumer's willingness to change lifestyle habits in the long term and orlistat is no different from other weight-loss aids in this respect. In fact because of its mode of action, orlistat encourages a change to less fatty foods that may help consumers to maintain a healthier lifestyle after stopping treatment.[16]

In the placebo-controlled studies, fewer subjects dropped out of the orlistat groups compared with the placebo groups and in a 'real-life' study, most subjects successfully maintained their diet while 32% increased the amount of exercise they took while taking orlistat.

The proposed indication for orlistat 60 mg does not include the use in children and adolescents under 18 years of age.

A pooled analysis of the data from the two pivotal studies of the original marketing authorization application demonstrated a similar efficacy of the 60 mg orlistat to that seen with 120 mg orlistat in patients with a BMI of 28 kg/m^2 or more (figure 14.1).

Based on the pooled analysis, the adjusted mean change from baseline after 6 months of treatment was −2.09 kg, −4.40 kg and −5.18 kg for placebo, 60 mg and 120 mg, respectively in the intent-to-treat population (ITT) population (p < 0.001 for the comparisons with placebo). There was some further weight loss in all three groups over the next 6 months of treatment. Adjusted mean change from baseline after 12 months of treatment was −2.32 kg, −4.78 kg and −5.56 kg for placebo, 60 mg and 120 mg, respectively, in the ITT population (p < 0.001 for the comparisons with placebo). Based on the comparison of the adjusted mean change from

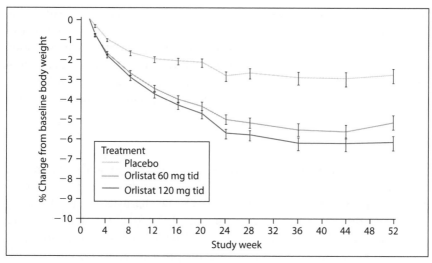

Figure 14.1 Relative change from baseline weight.

baseline for the 60-mg dose, 92% of the efficacy at 12 months was achieved at the 6-month timepoint.

A study of 'actual use' of orlistat 60 mg demonstrated an 80% customer satisfaction rate, alongside a median weight loss of around 5% after 60 days or more of use. Other, randomised, placebo-controlled studies showed a weight reduction of 50% more than diet and physical activity alone. Evidence shows that the use of orlistat 60 mg improves patterns of food purchases, suggesting a long-term commitment to healthy eating.

In a follow-up study, an overwhelming majority of subjects (>90%), indicated that they were very successful or somewhat successful in maintaining their diet. These results remained consistent at every interview for the duration of the study.

At study completion, approximately 32% of subjects indicated that they exercised more than they did prior to study enrolment.

Safety

Orlistat 120 mg has been on the market since 1998 and therefore there has been extensive patient exposure and there are no safety concerns. A number of studies have been completed with orlistat 60-mg capsules in the US and these provide further safety data for the product.

When any drug is switched to OTC there are always concerns that individuals who chose to use the product might take a higher dose than recommended. In studies there was no evidence of overdosing on 60 mg orlistat.

Drug interactions with orlistat are rare yet there exists a theoretical interaction between warfarin and orlistat based on orlistat's potential to reduce absorption of the fat-soluble vitamin K in the gut. One case of warfarin levels rising in a patient concomitantly taking orlistat has been reported in the US yet orlistat has been used widely across the world for a number of years and has been used in patients who are concomitantly using warfarin, yet post-marketing surveillance does not indicate a potential problem. Similarly, agents for other weight-related conditions, especially type 2 diabetes, may need adjusting as weight is lost, and it is important to liaise with general practice.

Pharmacist's role

In Europe orlistat will be restricted to pharmacy supply and therefore the pharmacist and pharmacy support staff will play a key role in the successful use of the product in managing obesity. Some pharmacists have derisively referred to orlistat as 'gastric Antabuse' or 'fried food punishment'. While this graphically describes the effect of orlistat, pharmacists can provide a more balanced explanation of orlistat for prospective users. Orlistat was never meant to be a weight-loss miracle – it is an aid to weight loss in patients who are already committed to becoming thinner. Such a patient will demonstrate that commitment, by voluntarily following a low-fat diet and exercising more, even prior to beginning therapy with orlistat.

Patients taking orlistat must commit to daily intake of a multivitamin containing beta-carotene and vitamins A, D, E, and K. As orlistat affects their absorption, failure to ingest them could lead to vitamin deficiencies, each with its well-known group of adverse effects.

Conclusion

There exists a huge market for a range of OTC slimming aids sold in the US and in Europe, mainly through pharmacies and health stores. With the exception of OTC orlistat, there exists very little evidence of efficacy for most of these products, and where efficacy does exist, there is the potential for adverse effects.

References

1. Krska J. OTC Slimming Aids. *Pharm J* 2008; 281: 181.
2. Maguire T. We are what we sell. *Pharm J* 2008; 281: 95.
3. Boon G, Lockwood B. *Pharm J* 2006; 276: 15–17.
4. Mason P. *Pharm J* 2002; 271: 103.
5. Pittler M, Ernst E. Dietary supplements for body weight reduction: a systematic review. *Am J Clin Nutr* 2004; 79: 529–536.
6. Hulisz D, Lindberg K. The skinny on weight loss supplements: fact or fantasy? http://cme.medscape.com/viewprogram/12613 (accessed 10 Jul 2009).
7. Shekelle P *et al.* Efficacy and safety of ephedra and ephedrine for weight loss and athletic performance. *JAMA* 2003; 289: 1537–1545.

8. Gades M D, Stern J S. Chitosan supplementation does not affect fat absorption in healthy males fed a high-fat diet, a pilot study. *Int J Obes* 2002; 26: 119–122.

9. Dixon J B. Weight loss medications – where do they fit in? *Aust Fam Phys* 2006; 35: 576–579.

10. Phytopharm plc. Hoodia factfile. Phytopharm 2006. Available at: http://www.phytopharm.com/hoodiafactfile (accessed 28 Mar 2008).

11. Villani R G *et al.* L-Carnitine supplementation combined with aerobic training does not promote weight loss in moderately obese women. *Int J Sport Nutr Exerc Metab* 2000; 10: 199–207.

12. Kovacs E M *et al.* Effects of green tea on weight maintenance after body-weight loss. *Br J Nutr* 2004; 91: 431–437.

13. Kriketos A D *et al.* (−)-Hydroxycitric acid does not affect energy expenditure and substrate oxidation in adult males in a post-absorptive state. *Int J Obes* 1999; 214: 867–873.

14. Anderson J W *et al.* Low-dose orlistat effects on body weight of mildly to moderately overweight individuals: a 16 week, double-blind, placebo-controlled trial. *Ann Pharmacother* 2006; 40: 1717–1723.

15. Schwartz S M *et al.* Compliance, behavior change and weight loss with orlistat in an over-the-counter setting. *Obesity* 2008; 16: 623–9.

16. Anderson J W. Orlistat for the management of overweight individuals and obesity: a review of potential for the 60-mg, over-the-counter dosage. *Expert Opin Pharmacother* 2007; 8: 1733–42.

Index

Note: page numbers in *italics* refer to boxes, figures and tables.